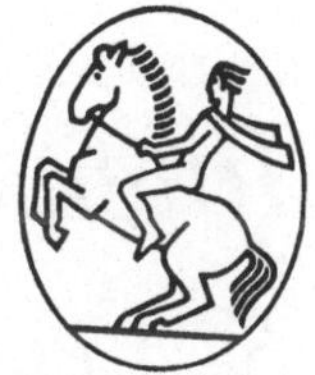

Intensivmedizinisches Seminar

K. Lenz, A. N. Laggner (Hrsg.)

Band 7

Springer-Verlag Wien New York

Metabolismus

*Stoffwechsel und Ernährung
kritisch kranker Patienten*

*(12. Wiener Intensivmedizinische Tage,
24.–26. Februar 1994)*

*G. Kleinberger, K. Lenz, R. Ritz,
B. Schneeweiß, H.-P. Schuster,
W. Waldhäusl (Hrsg.)*

Springer-Verlag Wien New York

Prof. Dr. Kurt Lenz, Wien
Prof. Dr. Anton N. Laggner, Wien

Prof. Dr. Gunther Kleinberger, Steyr
Prof. Dr. Kurt Lenz, Wien
Prof. Dr. Rudolf Ritz, Basel
Doz. Dr. Bruno Schneeweiß, Wien
Prof. Dr. Hans-Peter Schuster, Hildesheim
Prof. Dr. Werner Waldhäusl, Wien

Mit 29 Abbildungen

ISSN 0936-8507
ISBN-13: 978-3-211-82538-9   e-ISBN-13: 978-3-7091-9342-6
DOI: 10.1007/978-3-7091-9342-6

Vorwort

Störungen des Stoffwechsels stellen eines der zentralen Probleme in der Intensivmedizin dar. Hauptthema der 12. Wiener Intensivmedizinischen Tage war daher der Stoffwechsel kritisch kranker Patienten, deren wichtigste Vorträge im vorliegenden 7. Band des Intensivmedizinischen Seminars präsentiert werden. Dargestellt werden einerseits die pathophysiologischen Grundlagen des Energiestoffwechsels, andererseits die Möglichkeiten der optimalen Beeinflussung, soweit uns diese heute zur Verfügung stehen. Weiters wird auf spezielle Probleme bei einzelnen Erkrankungen, wie Sepsis, Schädelhirntrauma und ARDS eingegangen. Näher eingegangen wird weiters auf die Problematik des Energiestoffwechsels des beatmeten Patienten.

Insgesamt soll dieses Buch wiederum den Besuchern der Intensivmedizinischen Tage die Möglichkeit geben, Vorträge rasch zu rekapitulieren und eventuelle Unklarheiten zu klären.

Den Autoren sei wiederum sehr herzlich für die frühzeitige Bereitstellung ihrer Manuskripte gedankt. Nur durch ihre Mitarbeit war es möglich, auch heuer wiederum bereits zum Kongreß dieses Buch den Teilnehmern anbieten zu können.

Wien, im Jänner 1994   Die Herausgeber

Inhaltsverzeichnis

Nutrition of the critically ill: hypo, normo or hypercaloric

S. Bursztein

Rambam Medical Center, Technion-Israel Institute of Technology,
Haifa, Israel

To be fed is an absolute human right that should be given to all hospitalised patients, whom for a multitude of reasons may have difficulties in fulfilling this basic physiological function. In this category the critically ill and injured patients are at the forefront, usually unable to adequately feed themselves and with their increased energetic requirements, nutritional support must be provided artificially with the use of parenteral or enteral feeding techniques.

Although normal man has the fuel and nitrogen reserves enabling him to survive periods of fasting of up to 70 days [1, 2], injured, septic, traumatized and surgical patients usually have increased energy demands and higher rates of protein breakdown, decreasing their capacity to endure the added metabolic stress of starvation. Furthermore, it has been recognized that depleted patients irrespectively of their primary disease, have inadequate tissue repair mechanisms associated with depression of the immunity system. These abnormalities in synergism with those caused by the underlying disease render the stressed and/ or malnourished patient susceptible to an overhelming quantity of infectious complications which usually compromise the patient's survival. These observations are in accord with those of various other authors that demonstrate about half a century ago the increased incidence and severity of postoperative complications in patients who were protein deficient [3] or had lost more than 20 % of their total body weight [4].

These facts and the increased energy requirements have led to consider nutritional support as an essential part of the proper patient's management and especially the critically ill and injured.

In order to elucidate the modifications in energy requirements in the critically ill and injured patients and also how nutrients are utilized during artificial nutrition, we shall describe the energy metabolism patterns during a 24 hour period of fasting, during prolonged starvation and in hypermetabolic-hypercatabolic states.

Energy metabolism and substrate utilisation during fasting

We may consider that a normal 70 kg man has a pool of about 175,000 kcal, with mainly three types of fuel (carbohydrates, fat and proteins):

Table 1

Fat	16	kg	149,000 kcal
Proteins (mobilisable)	6	kg	24,000 kcal
Carbohydrates (Glycogen)	0,250	kg	1,000 kcal
Total			174,000 kcal

These stores, like stated before are theoretically sufficient for two months survival, for an individual utilising approximately 2500 kcal per day. A critically ill patient has an increased metabolic rate and will therefore deplete his stores in a shorter time. In the fasting situation, the body derives its energy only from its own stores of fat and glycogen as well as from functional intracellular proteins, mainly muscle proteins. During the first days, marked metabolic alterations occur, in order to conserve energy, but mainly to reduce protein breakdown; subsequent adaptations proceed at a slower rate.

After 24 hours of fasting, both liver and muscle retain some available glacogen, the actual amount depending on previous diet intake. Brain glucose requirements are much greater than the amounts that can be supplied by the body stores, and the rest is obtained from gluconeogenesis in the liver, using amino acids, primarily from breakdown of muscle protein, but also glycerol derived from lipolysis of adipose tissue triglycerides. Lactate and pyruvate, produced by red and white cells and other glycolizing tissues such as the kidney medulla and lens of the eye, are also substrates for glucose production in the liver [5].

The brain also obtains a small amount of energy from oxidation of ketone bodies even at this early stage of fasting. It was formerly thought that the brain had to adapt to oxidation of ketone bodies, but it is now clear that the proportions of glucose and ketone bodies utilized by the brain depend on their relative concentrations in the blood. After prolonged starvation, ketone body concentrations are higher than those of glucose, and they provide more than one half of brain energy requirements. When ketone bodies concentrations reach high levels, substantial amounts are excreted in the urine, and fasting of more than 3 or 4 days is associated with metabolic acidosis. In normal subjects as well as in hypercatabolic states most of the nitrogen is excreted in the urine in the form of urea, but in prolonged fasting there is a remarkable protein sparing effect decreasing protein breakdown and in the same time the nitogen excreted in the urine has a relative lower proportion of urea and a larger proportion of ammonium, wich corrects partly the metabolic acidosis by excreting H^+ ions. The weights and intracellular Nitrogen (N) contents of all organs and tissues, decrease during fasting or starvation, except for the brain and nervous tissue which show negligible changes.

After 4 or 5 days of fasting, available glycogen stores are completely depleted, and glucose and insulin concentrations are at minimum levels. An increasing portion of gluconeogenesis takes place in the kidney.

In fasting, the brain minimizes glucose oxidation, replacing it with ketone bodies oxidation and this adaptation permits a reduction in protein breakdown from about 75 g, in the beginning of the fasting period, to about 20 g/day after several weeks. This is reflected in a sensible decrease in urea excretion.

Energy metabolism and substrate utilisation during hypermetabolic states

The injured, traumatized or septic patient is hypermetabolic, hypercatabolic, has increased fat mobilization and oxidation and is glucose and insulin resistant [6]. Nitrogen excretion is more than twice normal and can reach up to 600 mg/kg/day in patients receiving 5 % dextrose solutions.

These metabolic changes cause the critically ill patient to have increased nutrient requirements, which must be obtained from body stores. Various authors have suggested that the increased muscle protein breakdown is needed as a major source of energy in these patients. However, in severe stress, it has been observed that endogenous protein accounts for less than 25 % of total energy requirements [7].

Furthermore, mobilization of fat, which is the major endogenous source of fuel, is greatly increased with stress. It seems more likely that the increased muscle proteolysis is needed to supply specific nutrients, glucose and amino acids (AA), which cannot be derived from fat. This increased source of AA is required for synthesis of acute phase proteins and white blood cells needed for the control of infection, the clearing of necrotic tissue and wound healing. In addition, in the absence of endogenous carbohydrates stores, AA are the main source for synthesis of the glucose needed by the brain and other glucose requiring tissues, particularly the wound and the white blood cells.

In severe burns it has been demonstrated that the wound itself may require up to 200 g of glucose per day [8]. However, interestingly, the wound does not oxidize the glucose but obtains its energy from anaerobic glycolysis. Since glucose is not oxidized but converted to lactate which is largely used for resynthesis of glucose in the liver there is little or no net requirement of glucose by the wound. Nevertheless, this enormous requirement of the wound for glucose, as well as the insulin resistance, seems the most likely explanation for the hyperglycemia assoicated with severe injury.

Energy balance

The concept of energy balance is very simple:

$$\text{Energy balance} = \text{energy in} - \text{energy out}$$

If "energy in" equals "energy out", the subject is in zero energy balance.

If "energy in" is greater than "energy out", the subject is in positive energy balance and is storing energy mainly as fat. If "energy out" is greater than "energy in", the subject is in negative energy balance and must be oxidizing endogenous stores of energy, again mainly fat.

Energy intake is equal to the sum of the caloric intaktes of fat, carbohydrate and protein and, when applicable alcohol. The most accurate method for measuring energy intake is to determine the energy of the food eaten by a bomb calorimeter. However, when using chemically defined diets for tube feeding, or dextrose, amino acid solutions and lipid emulsions for parenteral nutrition, the procedure is greatly simplified and improves the accuracy of intake estimates.

There are nevertheless a number of problems that must be kept in mind:

1) Caloric content of dextrose, which is glucose monohydrate, is 3.41 kcal/g, and is not the same as that of glucose, 3.75 kcal/g, or of starch which is 4.17 kcal/g. Thus the energy content of 1 liter of 5 % dextrose solution ist 170 kcal and not 200 kcal which is often used in clinical literature.

2) The energy constants to be used with parenteral solutions are the gross energy constants, not the metabolizable constants, since there is no intestinal loss of these nutrients. With enteral solutions there may be losses due to lack of absorbtion.

3) The contents as listed by the manufacturer may not be correct, however, such variations are not important for clinical monitoring, but may be important for research studies. We may conclude that without due precautions and sophisticated equipment errors of 10 % or greater are usual in calculating energy intake.

Energy expenditure (EE) in a clinical setting is most accurately determined by the measurements of oxygen consumption (VO_2) and carbon dioxide production (VCO_2) by the indirect calorimetry method. Bedside metabolic carts and monitors are today readily available for measuring VO_2 and VCO_2, and with one measurement of 15 to 20 minutes an evaluation of daily EE can be obtained with an error not greater than 10 %. However, in the absence of such equipment resting energy expenditure (REE) may be estimated for normal subjects, with less than 10 %

error from the formulas of Harris and Benedict based on height, weight, age and sex.

The Harris and Benedict formulae are:

For men: REE(kcal/day) = 66.5 + 13.75 W + 5.0 H − 6.76 A

For women: REE(kcal/day) = 655.1 + 9.56 W + 1.85 H − 4.67 A

Where: W = weight (kg), H = height (cm), A = age (years)

If acceptable estimates of REE may be made from these formulae in normals, when measurement devices are not available, corrections are necessary and not always reliable for the degree of stress and/or malnutrition in the critically ill. Increases in REE are approximately 10 % to 20 % for elective surgery, 20 to 50 % for accidental injury, 20 to 60 % for sepsis and up to 100 % for severe burns [9]. Malnutrition on the other hand may decrease REE by 40 % while provision of adequate nutrient intake will increase REE by 10 to 30 % above that seen during 5 % dextrose infusion alone [10]. Frequently ICU patients may combine all these factors resulting in highly variable REE which can change markedly from day to day. Therefore, direct measurement of EE by indirect calorimetry is essential in acutely ill patients in order to correctly determine the magnitude of their energy expenditure.

Nitrogen balance

Like for energy balance the concept of nitrogene balance is:

Nitrogen Balance = nitrogen in − nitrogen out

If "nitrogen in" equals "nitrogren out", the subject is in zero nitrogen balance. If "nitrogen in" is greater than "nitrogen out", the subject is in positive nitrogen balance. If "nitrogen out" is greater that "nitrogen in", the subject is in negative nitrogen balance. Nitrogen (N) balance is a complex function of protein breakdown and both energy and N intakes. When N intake is kept constant, increasing energy intake will increase N balance to the point where N intake becomes limiting and further increases in energy intake will have no positive effect on N balance. At low energy intakes this effect is large, about 7 mg N for each additional kcal, and is seen mainly with carbohydrate and much less with fat. Above one-half energy requirements, the effect on N balance is much smaller, about 2 mg N per kcal and is shared by fat.

Increasing N intake will also increase N balance as long as energy intake does not become limiting. However, well nourished adults will not attain positive N balance, at any reasonable level of N intake, as long as they are at zero energy balance. Positive N balance can be achieved in healthy adults only by providing energy in excess of requirements. In this condition the increase of fat deposition, will necessitate the neoformation of a proteic structure and of new vessels. On the other hand, nutritionally depleted adults can reach positive N balance at zero or even negative energy balance if N intake is high enough. It follows that N balance in malnourished patients can be increased by increasing either energy or N intakes. In sufficiently severe stress it is impossible to achieve zero N balance at any N intake even though energy is supplied in higher amounts than energy expenditure.

In order to restore tissue in these conditions it is necessary to provide very high N intakes while keeping energy intakes above energy expenditure.

This does not solve the problem of how much calories have to be given when the EE is known. Should nutrition be Hypo, normo or hypercaloric.

Hypo, normo or hypercaloric nutrition for the critically ill

The changed neuroendocrine milieu in stressed patients changes the response to nutrients. Since fuel utilization patterns are now largely determined by the increased sympathetic activity and counterregulatory hormones, the ability of exogenous nutrients, particularly glucose, to change these patterns is attenuated.

In septic or injured patients receiving 3 liters of 5 % dextrose, gluconeogenesis is twice as high as in fasting normal subjects. Even with glucose intakes in excess of energy expenditure, the injured and septic patients derived one third of their energy from endogenous fat.

The effect of protein intake to imprive N balance is attenuated injured, septic or burned patients. Normal subjects attain zero N balance at zero energy balance with an intake of 80 mg N/kg/day, whereas severely stressed patients are in negative N balance of 3–4 g per day with N intakes of 200 to 300 mg/kg/ day and energy intake in excess of expenditure.

Nutritional problems arise in the critically ill when they are unable to receive adequate nutrients by oral intake. The major problems in determing optimal amounts of essential nutrient administration concern the macronutrients, carbohydrate, fat and protein. Nevertheless, it is imperative to emphasize that maintenance and regulation of body cell mass (BCM) requires adequate intake of all other essential nutrients provided for the most part on a daily basis. For instance, omission from an otherwise adequate diet of either potassium (K), phosphate (P), or nitrogen (N) will convert markedly positive N and K balances to negative within one day.

The requirement for fat is essentially a requirement for the dietary essential fatty acid, linoleic acid of about 10 g/day. This is usually met by administration of 200 ml of a 10 % fat emulsion which is approximately equal to 10 % of total energy require- ments. As for the other essential fatty acid, linolenic acid, the daily requirement is not presently known.

There is no absolute requirement for carbohydrate in the diet since it can be synthesized from protein or to a limited extent from fat. However, there is a requirement for glucose by the brain and nervous tissue which comprises 20 % of REE. In the absence of carbohydrate this can be met by providing 200 g protein/day, but is much better met by providing every day 100– 150 g carbohydrate. Injured or septic patients are glucose and insulin resistant and may require larger amounts. Therefore, at least 25 % of REE should be provided as carbohydrate and in stressed patients this has to be increased. However, both car- bohydrate and protein have marked effects on respiration. The respiratory quotient (RQ) for carbohydrate oxidation is 1.0, while the RQ for fat is 0.71 and that for protein is about 0.80.

Administration of hypercaloric glucose based TPN can raise the RQ as high as 1.2, and at the same time can cause a doubling of CO_2 production and a corresponding increase in minute ven- tilation (VE). Protein or amino acid infusion cause an increase in respiratory response or sensitivity to CO_2, so that administra- tion of too much protein adds to the respiratory effects of car- bohydrate. For patients with inadequate pulmonary reserve this may induce respiratory distress and prevent weaning from respirators.

In patients lacking pulmonary reserve, carbohydrate intake should be kept between 25 and 50 % of REE. For previously well nourished subjects who have suffered injury, burns, or elective surgery or who are septic, the goals of nutritional therapy are to prevent, maintain or minimize losses of lean body mass (LBM). Since in severely stressed patients N losses can reach between 15–40 g/day, full enteral or parenteral nutrition is justified and should be provided if the patient is not expected to return to adequate oral intake within a day or two. Nutritional requirements should be met but not be much in excess of energy expenditure and should provide about 200 mg N/kg/day. Although zero N balance may not be achieved, administration of more N will have little effect. Furthermore, since these patients are resistant particularly to glucose, non protein energy should be provided as equal amounts of both fat and carbohydrate. When the patients status ameliorates and become less hypermetabolic and hypercatabolic, both energy and N intakes can be increased to recuperate previous losses.

A particularly difficult problem is posed in the nutritional support of severely stressed patients who are also malnourished. In these patients it is probably impossible to maintain, much less to restore LBM and nutritional support is instituted with the only hope of minimizing losses, at least at the begin of treatment.

A lot of studies were performed to establish the ideal amounts of nutrients to be administered in critically ill, since total parenteral nutrition (TPN) was instituted by Dudrick in the end of the sixties. At this time, many critically ill patients probably survived thanks to this treatment, although they were receiving twice or three times their energy expenditure. Then, since intravenous lipid emulsions were not available, several publications showed that high amounts of carbohydrate intake produces fatty liver, and caloric supply was considerably reduced. In the last decade, energy expenditure is more and more measured in intensive care, and the general accepted approach is to administer between 25 % to 50 % more calories, than the expended amounts, which is less than hypercaloric, but more than hypo or normocaloric.

References

1. Bursztein S, Elwyn DH, Askanazi, et al (1989) The theoretical framework of indirect calorimetry and energy balance. In: Energy metabolism, indirect calorimetry and nutrition. Williams and Wilkins, Baltimore
2. Gamble JL (1947) Physiological information gained from studies on the life raft ration. Harvey Lect 42: 247–273
3. Cannon PR, Wissler RW, Woolridge RL, et al (1944) The relationship of protein deficiency to surgical infection. Ann Surg 120: 514–521
4. Studley HO (1936) Percentage of weighy loss: a basic indicator of surgical risk in patients with chronic peptic ulcer. JAMA 106: 458–462
5. Cahil GF Jr (1970) Starvation in man. N Engl J Med 282: 668–675
6. Elwyn DH, Kinney JM, Jeevanandam M, et al (1979) Influence of increasing carbohydrate intake on glucose kinetics in injured patients. Ann Surg 190: 117–127
7. Kinney JM, Elwyn DH (1983) Protein metabolism and injury. Ann Rev Nutr 3: 433–466
8. Wilmore DW, Aulick LH (1978) Metabolic changes in burned patients. Surg Clin North Am 58: 1173–1187
9. Kinney JM, Duke JH, Jr, Long CL, et al (1970) Tissue fuel and weight loss after injury. J Clin Pathol [Suppl 4]: 65–72
10. Acheson KJ, Schutz Y, Bessard T, Ravussen E, Jerquier E (1984) Nutritional influences on lipogenesis and thermogenesis after a carbohydrate meal. Am J Physiol 246: E62–E67

Correspondence: Prof. Dr. S. Bursztein, Director, Intensive Care Department, Rambam Medical Center, Technion – Israel Institute of Technology, Haifa, Israel

Die Bedeutung der Messung des Sauerstofftransportes und Sauerstoffverbrauches beim Intensivpatienten

B. Schneeweiß

Intensivstation, Klinik für Innere Medizin IV,
Universität Wien, Österreich

Physiologische Reaktionsmöglichkeiten auf Änderungen des Sauerstoffangebotes

Biologische Systeme (Zellen, Gewebe, Lebewesen) deren Sauerstoffverbrauch (VO_2) eine Abhängigkeit von Sauerstoffangebot [z. B. ausgedrückt durch den Sauerstofftransport (DO_2)] in einem weiten Bereich zeigt, werden als *O₂-conformers* bezeichnet. Ist der VO_2 hingegen weitgehend unabhängig vom DO_2 sprechen wir von *O₂-regulators* [1]. Der Skelettmuskel ist ein typischer Vertreter der Gruppe der O₂-conformers: ein VO_2-Plateau kann selbst für sehr hohe DO_2-Werte kaum erreicht werden (Abb. 1). Mitochondrien und das Säugetiergehirn zeigen hingegen die typischen Charakteristika eines O₂-regulators: die Respiration, d. h. der VO_2 sind weitgehend unabhängig vom O₂-Angebot (Abb. 2). Der O₂-Verbrauch der Leber und auch der Gesamt-O₂-Verbrauch des Menschen zeigen eine Abhängigkeit vom DO_2, die zwischen derjenigen eines typischen O₂-conformers und O₂-regulators liegt: der VO_2 zeigt bis zu einem kritischen Wert keine Abhängigkeit vom DO_2, erst unterhalb dieses „kritischen DO_2" findet sich das Bild wie bei einem O₂-conformers (Abb. 3). Dieser kritische DO_2 wird bei gesunden Menschen mit 330 ml/min. m² bzw. 8–10 ml/min. kg angegeben [2].

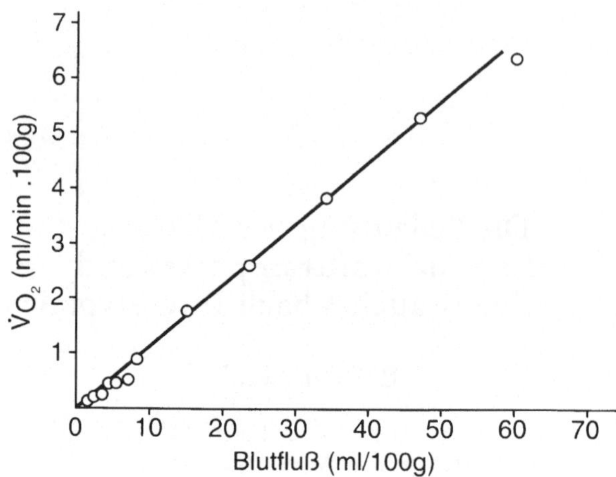

Abb. 1. Beziehung zwischen Sauerstofftransport (Blutfluß) und Sauerstoffverbrauch ($\dot{V}O_2$) im Skelettmuskel als Beispiel eines O_2-conformers

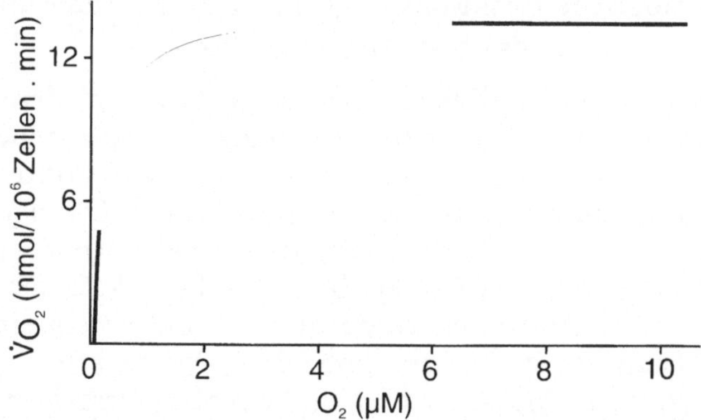

Abb. 2. $\dot{V}O_2$-O_2-Konzentrationsbeziehung bei O_2-regulators
(z. B. Mitochondrien)

Die weitgehende Unabhängigkeit des $\dot{V}O_2$ vom DO_2
oberhalb dieses kritischen DO_2 wird durch Variationen in der
Sauerstoffextraktion gewährleistet [3]: bei einer Reduktion des
DO_2 nimmt die Sauerstoffextraktion zu, um beim kritischen
DO_2 ein Maximum zu erreichen. Diese Parameter weisen
allerdings eine Gewebsabhängigkeit auf, wobei besonders der
Darm eine deutlich niedrigere kritische Sauerstoffextraktionsrate
zeigt [4].

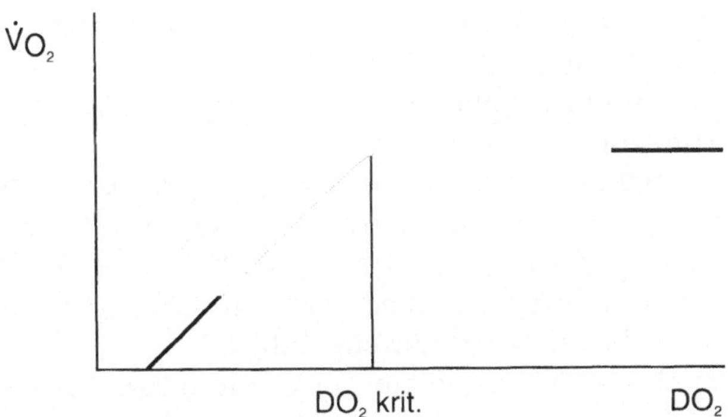

Abb. 3. Charakteristische Beziehung zwischen VO_2 und Sauerstoffangebot (DO_2) beim Menschen. DO_2 krit ~ 330 ml/min m²

Veränderungen der VO_2-DO_2-Korrelation bei kritisch kranken Patienten (Die pathologische DO_2-Abhängigkeit)

Bei Patienten mit ARDS und Sepsis konnte eine DO_2-Abhängigkeit des VO_2 schon bei normalen und auch bei hohen DO_2-Werten gefunden werden (= pathologische DO_2-Korrelation). Der kritische DO_2 beträgt bei diesen Patienten >15–20 ml/min kg [5, 6]. Als Ursache wird ein eingeschränktes Sauerstoffextraktionsvermögen der peripheren Gewebe diskutiert [3]. Zudem findet sich bei diesen Krankheitsbildern ein gesteigerter VO_2, welcher per se zu einer Erhöhung des kritischen DO_2 führt.

Da nun bei diesen Zustandsbildern erhöhte arterielle Laktatkonzentrationen gefunden werden konnten und zudem diese Patienten eine deutlich erhöhte Mortalität aufweisen [7], wird eine pathologische DO_2-Abhängigkeit häufig als Indikator für das Vorliegen einer Gewebshypoxie angesehen [7].

Bestimmung der Korrelation VO_2-DO_2 („oxygen flux Test")

VO_2 und DO_2 werden in der klinischen Praxis mit Hilfe des Fickschen Prinzips unter Zuhilfenahme eines Pulmonaliskatheters bestimmt:

DO_2 = Herzminutenvolumen $\times$ arterielle Sauerstoffkonzentration

VO_2 = Herzminutenvolumen $\times$ arterio-venöse Sauerstoffkonzentrationsdifferenz

Im Rahmen des sogenannten „oxygen-flux" Testes wird nun beurteilt, inwieweit eine Steigerung des DO_2 zu einer Erhöhung des VO_2 führt [7]. Die Variation des DO_2 wird durch Volumengabe, durch Katecholamine, bzw. andere vasoaktive Substanzen (z. B. Prostacyclin) durchgeführt.

Ein methodisches Problem muß allerdings berücksichtigt werden, wenn DO_2 und VO_2 mit Hilfe des Fickschen Prinzips bestimmt werden. Unter diesen Bedingungen besteht die Möglichkeit einer „mathematischen Kopplung" beider Meßgrößen: das Herzminutenvolumen stellt eine gemeinsame Variable in der Berechnung von VO_2 und DO_2 dar. Ein Meßfehler in bezug auf das Herzminutenvolumen kann dadurch eine Korrelation zwischen beiden Parametern vortäuschen und zu falschen Konklusionen Anlaß geben [8]. Aus diesen Gründen wäre zu fordern, daß VO_2 und DO_2 unabhängig voneinander bestimmt werden, DO_2 mit Hilfe des oben beschriebenen Fickschen Prinzips, VO_2 mit Hilfe der indirekten Kalorimetrie. Letztgenannte Technik liefert allerdings bei maschinell beatmeten Patienten mit einem FIO_2 >0,4 aus methodischen Gründen keine zuverlässigen Daten.

Stellt eine „pathologische" VO_2-DO_2-Korrelation einen Hinweis auf das Vorliegen einer Gewebshypoxie dar?

Diese Frage wurde von Cain und Curtis treffend folgendermaßen formuliert: *„Is supply truly limiting VO_2 or is an increase in supply actually driving VO_2?"* [3]. Diese Frage ist insbesondere dann von Bedeutung, wenn die Erhöhung des DO_2 durch Katecholaminmedikation bedingt ist, da dadurch auch direkt der VO_2 gesteigert wird [9].

Hinweise dafür, daß unter den Bedingungen einer pathologischen VO_2-DO_2-Korrelation eine Gewebshypoxie vorliegt, sind die bei septischen Patienten und beim ARDS gemachten Beobachtungen einer Störung des Sauerstofftransport zu den Zellen und zu den Mitochondrien. Diese Beeinträchtigung des Sauerstofftransportes ist durch Veränderungen in der Mikrozirkulation bedingt (Mikrothromben, perikapilläres Ödem, Störung der funktionellen Regulation der Mikrozirkulation) [10]. Eine Erhöhung des kapillären Sauerstoffangebotes würde unter diesen Bedingungen zweifellos eine vorliegende Gewebshypoxie beseitigen.

Die bei septischen Patienten wiederholt beobachteten erhöhten arteriellen Laktatkonzentrationen könnten ebenfalls als Indikator für das Vorliegen einer Gewebshypoxie gewertet werden [11]. In der letzten Zeit mehren sich allerdings die Hinweise, daß erhöhte Blutlaktatkonzentrationen in der Sepsis und ARDS nicht so sehr im Sinne einer Gewebshypoxie zu interpretieren als vielmehr durch eine Inaktivierung des Enzyms Pyruvatdehydrogenase bedingt sind [3]. Eine Hemmung dieses Enzyms würde die Glukoseoxidationsrate vermindern und dadurch zu einer gesteigerten Fett- und Proteinoxidation führen; dies sind Veränderungen des Substratstoffwechsels wie sie bei septischen Patienten beobachtet werden [12]. Darüber hinaus konnte in vitro gezeigt werden, daß Endotoxin eine Inaktivierung der Pyruvatdehydrogenase bewirkt [13]. Erhöhte Laktatspiegel können somit auch Ausdruck nicht hypoxisch bedingter metabolischer Konsequenzen der Sepsis sein. Der Quotient aus Laktat/Pyruvat scheint zur Diagnose einer Gewebshypoxie besser geeignet zu sein: Nicht durch eine Gewebshypoxie bedingte Erhöhungen der arteriellen Laktatkonzentration zeigen eine ähnlich ausgeprägte Erhöhung der Pyruvatkonzentration, sodaß das Konzentrationsverhältnis beider Substrate zueinander unverändert bleibt. Ein Anstieg dieses Quotienten (d. h. Laktat > Pyruvat) würde hingegen für eine Gewebshypoxie sprechen [14].

Zusammenfassung

Bei Patienten mit ARDS/Sepsis findet sich eine Abhängigkeit des VO_2 vom DO_2 schon in supranormalen DO_2-Bereichen. Diese „pathologische" VO_2-DO_2 Korrelation wird üblicherweise als Hinweis für das Vorliegen einer Gewebshypoxie gewertet. Methodische und physiologische Argumente sprechen allerdings gegen diese Interpretation. Auch die bei pathologischen VO_2-DO_2-Korrelationen häufig erhöhten Laktatkonzentrationen können nicht als eindeutiger Hypoxieindikator gewertet werden.

Da die Reaktion auf eine Hypoxie (O_2-regulators, O_2-conformers) und die kritischen DO_2-Werte in verschiedenen Geweben unterschiedlich sind, müssen Messungen des Gesamt-O_2 und -DO_2 mit Vorsicht interpretiert werden. Die Bedeutung der Messung des O_2-Transportes und O_2-Verbrauches beim Intensivpatienten für die klinische Praxis kann somit zur Zeit noch nicht klar beurteilt werden.

Literatur

1. Hochachka PW, Guppy M (1987) Metabolic arrest and the control of biological time. Harvard University Press, Cambridge, pp 10–35
2. Shibutani K, Komatsu T, Kubal K, et al (1983) Critical level of oxygen delivery in anesthetized man. Crit Care Med 11: 640
3. Cain SM, Curtis SE (1991) Experimental models of pathologic oxygen supply dependency. Crit Care Med 19: 603
4. Nelson DP, Samsel RW, Wood LDH, et al (1988) Pathologic supply dependence of systemic and intestinal oxygen uptake during endotoxemia. J Appl Physiol 64: 2410
5. Mohsenifar Z, Goldbach P, Tashkin DP, et al (1983) Relationship between O_2 delivery and O_2 consumption in the adult respiratory distress syndrome. Chest 84: 267
6. Tuchschmidt J, Oblitas D, Fried JC (1991) Oxygen consumption in sepsis and septic shock. Crit Care Med 19: 664
7. Bihari D, Smithies M, Gimson A, et al (1987) The effects of vasodilation with prostacyclin on oxygen delivery and uptake in critically ill patients. N Engl J Med 317: 397
8. Vermeij CG, Feenstra BWA, Bruining HA (1990) Oxygen delivery and oxygen uptake in postoperative and septic patients. Chest 98: 415
9. Staten MA, Matthews DE, Cryer PE, et al (1987) Physiological increments in epinephrine stimulate metabolic rate in humans. Am J Physiol 253: E322
10. Cain SM (1986) Assessment of tissue oxygenation. Crit Care Clin 2: 537
11. Weg JG (1991) Oxygen transport in adult respiratory distress syndrome and other acute circulatory problems: relationship of oxygen delivery and oxygen consumption. Crit Care Med 19: 650
12. Cerra FB (1987) Hypermetabolism, organ failure, and metabolic support. Surgery 101: 1
13. Kilpatrick-Smith L, Erecinska M (1983) Cellular effects of endotoxin in vitro. I. Effect of endotoxin on mitochondrial substrate metabolism and intracellular calcium. Circ Shock 11: 85

14. Huckabee WE (1958) Relationships of pyruvate and lactate during anaerobic metabolism. I. Effects of infusion of pyruvate or glucose and of hyperventilation. J Clin Invest 37: 244

Korrespondenz: Univ.-Doz. Dr. B. Schneeweiß, Intensivstation 13 H1, Klinik für Innere Medizin IV, Universität Wien, Währinger Gürtel 18–20, A-1090 Wien, Österreich

Der Einfluß der Temperatur auf den Stoffwechsel

M. Hiesmayr, P. Keznickl, D. Heilinger, A. Lassnigg, P. Mares,
H. Steltzer, M. Semsroth und W. Haider

Abteilung für Herz-Thorax-Gefäßanästhesie und Intensivmedizin und
Abteilung für Allgemeine Anästhesie und Intensivmedizin,
Klinik für Anästhesie und Allgemeine Intensivmedizin, Universität Wien,
Österreich

Während der amerikanische Alligator als Wechselblüter lediglich
60 Kcal/24 h bei einer Umgebungstemperatur von 20° C an
Wärme produziert [1], verbrennt der Mensch bei der gleichen
Umgebungstemperatur 1800 Kcal/24 h, um seine Körpertemperatur auf 37° C konstant zu halten. Drei physiologische
Gründe werden für dieses Verhalten genannt [12].

1. Ein konstantes Temperaturmilieu ist für viele Zellen vorteilhaft [61] und erlaubt eine adäquate Funktion des Gesamtorganismus unabhängig von der thermischen Umwelt.

2. Um überschüssige Wärme, wie sie bei körperlicher Aktivität entsteht, leicht loswerden zu können, muß die Körpertemperatur möglichst hoch über der durchschnittlichen Umgebungstemperatur (22° C gesamte Erde) liegen.

3. Das Zentralnervensystem (ZNS) ist funktionell eingeschränkt unter 35° C und über 40,5° C treten irreversible
Schäden auf.

Die Körpertemperatur wird beim Menschen in einem extrem
engen Bereich (±0,3° C) [38] bei intaktem Nervensystem geregelt. Dabei spielen neben physiologischen Antworten auch
Verhaltensänderungen eine entscheidende Rolle (Abb. 1). Wenn
die gesamte Temperaturregulation nur durch Änderungen des
Energieumsatzes (EE) möglich wäre [29], wäre das Ziel der Un-

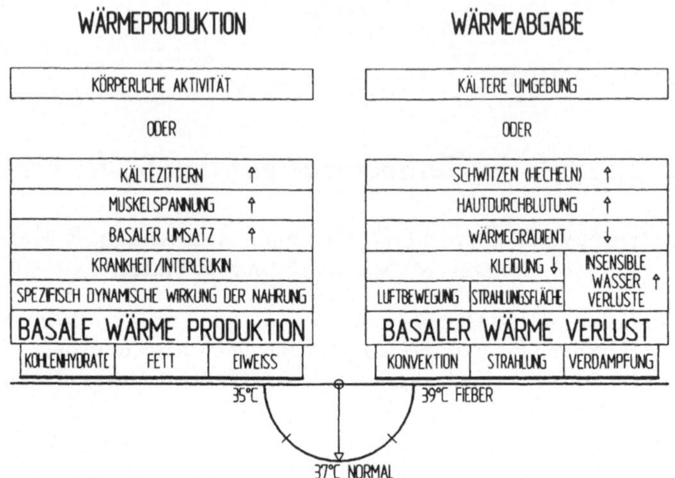

Abb. 1. Diagramm des thermischen Gleichgewichts und der Faktoren von Wärmeproduktion und Wärmeverlust

abhängigkeit stark eingeschränkt und die Regulation sehr ineffektiv und unökonomisch.

Der kritische Kranke auf der Intensivstation ist nicht mehr in der Lage auf die ökonomischen Mechanismen der Verhaltensanpassung zurückzugreifen und ist in seiner Stoffwechselleistung auch der Dynamik der Erkrankung und Therapie unterworfen. Diese Übersicht soll die Physiologie, Pathophysiologie und mögliche Therapie der Wechselwirkung von Körpertemperatur und Stoffwechsel untersuchen.

Messung von Temperatur und Stoffwechsel

Obwohl seit 1611 (Sanctorius) Temperaturmessungen durchgeführt wurden, ist die routinemäßige Messung der Körpertemperatur erst seit 1870 allgemein angewandt worden. Die Kerntemperatur kann am besten in der Pulmonalarterie gemessen werden, jedoch können vergleichbare Werte in der Blase eventuell im Rektum oder im Mund gemessen werden [20]. Auf erhebliche Schwierigkeiten stößt man, wenn man die mittlere Körpertemperatur messen möchte.

Die Messung des Energieumsatzes (EE) bzw. der Wärmeproduktion ist erst viel jüngeren Datums. Die direkte Kalorimetrie wurde kurz vor Beginn des 20. Jahrhunderts eingeführt [3]. Diese Methode ist mit einem Fehler von 1 % bei Messungen über mehrere Stunden sehr exakt, erlaubt aber keine externen Manipulationen der Wärmebilanz (Abb. 1) und ist klinisch nicht einsetzbar. Kurz davor wurde von Pettenkofer [40] der Grundstein für die indirekte Kalorimetrie gesetzt, wobei Pflüger die theoretischen Grundlagen erarbeitete [41]. Mittels respiratorischer indirekter Kalorimetrie wird die Sauerstoffaufnahme ($V'O_2$) und die Kohlendioxidabgabe ($V'CO_2$) mit einer Genauigkeit von 5 % gemessen. Als große Einschränkung erweist sich die Unmöglichkeit einer exakten Messung bei FiO_2 > 0,6–0,7. Die mittels unterschiedlicher Formeln berechneten Stoffwechselumsätze (Tabelle 1) sind schon mit Unterschieden von 5–8 % behaftet. Die Vernachlässigung der Stickstoffausscheidung bewirkt lediglich eine Fehlbewertung von 4 %. Falls keine respiratorische indirekte Kalorimetrie zur Verfügung steht kann man sich mittels zirkulatorischer indirekter Kalori-

Tabelle 1. Formeln zur Berechnung des Energieumsatzes (EE) in Kcal/24 h aus Sauerstoffverbrauch ($V'O_2$) in ml/min, Kohlendioxidproduktion ($V'CO_2$) in ml/min und Stickstoffausscheidung N' in g/24 h. Umrechnung von ml/min auf Liter/24 h durch den Faktor 1.44

Respiratorische indirekte Kalorimetrie

EE	24 h	$V'O_2$	$V'CO_2$	N'	Bemerkung	Literatur
EE =	1.44x	(3.940 $V'O_2$ + 1.110 $V'CO_2$	−2.17 N'			[58]
EE =	1.44x	(3.796 $V'O_2$ + 1.214 $V'CO_2$)				[53], [58]
EE =	1.44x	(3.940 $V'O_2$ + 1.100 $V'CO_2$)			Schädelhirntrauma	[9], [60]
EE =	1.44x	(3.810 $V'O_2$ + 1.14 $V'CO_2$)	corr N'		nüchtern	[30]
EE =	1.44x	(5.120 $V'O_2$ − 0.17 $V'CO_2$)			postabsorptiv	[30]
EE =	1.44x	(3.780 $V'O_2$ + 1.160 $V'CO_2$)	+2.98 N'		nonprotein RQ< 1	[10]
EE =	1.44x	(5.083 $V'O_2$ + 0.138 $V'CO_2$)	−0.128 N'		nonprotein RQ> 1	[10]
EE =	1.44x	(3.581 $V'O_2$ + 1.448 $V'CO_2$)	−32.4		nüchtern	[33]

Zirkulatorische indirekte Kalorimetrie

EE =	1.44x 4.860 $V'O_2$	[8, 36, 60]

metrie behelfen, wobei mit Fehlern bei der Berechnung des V'O$_2$ von 10–15 % und bei der Berechnung des EE von 15–20 % gerechnet werden muß. Außerdem wurden systematisch niedrigere Werte (16–24 %) gemessen [55], welche zum Teil mit der Vernachlässigung des V'O$_2$ der Lunge erklärt wurden.

Umgebungstemperatur und Stoffwechsel beim Gesunden

Die Anpassung der Stoffwechselrate an die Außentemperatur ist in Abb. 2 schematisch dargestellt. In der thermisch neutralen Zone ist die basale Stoffwechselrate (BMR = basal metabolic rate) beim Erwachsenen 60–70 Kcal/h (70–80 Watt). Wenn die

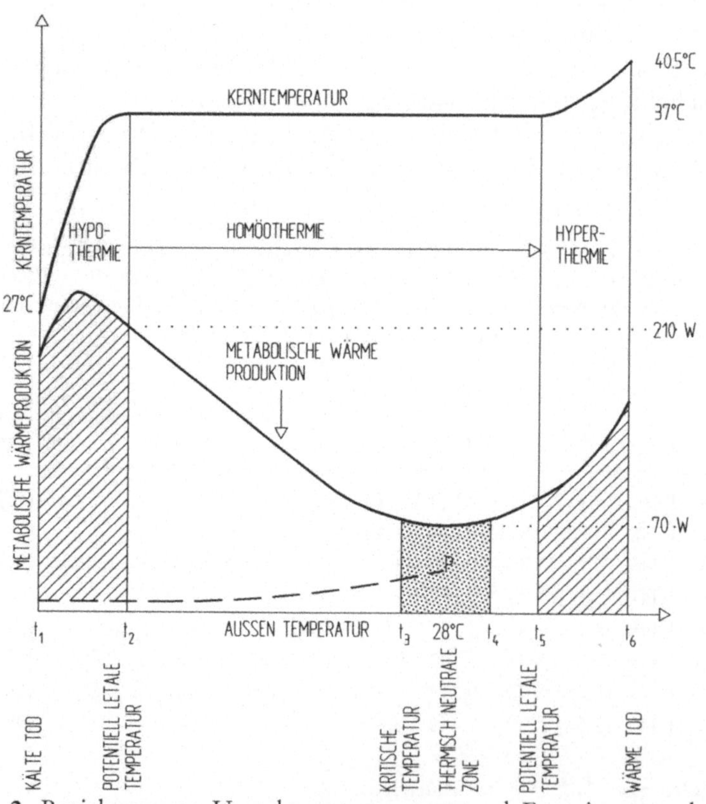

Abb. 2. Beziehung von Umgebungstemperatur und Energieumsatz beim Menschen

thermisch neutrale Zone te$_3$-t$_4$ (um 28° C) verlassen wird, steigt die Stoffwechselrate an.

Wenn t$_4$ überschritten wird, beginnt die Stoffwechselrate rasch anzusteigen. Aufgrund der Eigenschaften der Enzyme ändert sich die Reaktionsgeschwindigkeit um einen Faktor 2–3 pro 10° C Temperaturänderung. Diese Änderung mit der Temperatur ist stärker, als bei rein chemischen Reaktionen. Gleichzeitig setzt die Gegenregulation in Form von Vasodilatation und Schwitzen ein. Wenn die Kerntemperatur 40,5° C erreicht, ist der einzige Schutz des Gehirns ein maximaler Blutfluß in den Venen der Kopfhaut, der es vermag die Temperatur des einströmenden Blutes in der A. carotis gering zu senken [13].

Wenn t$_3$ unterschritten wird, stellt die Steigerung der Stoffwechselrate eine sinnvolle Gegenregulation dar. Sie erreicht ihr Maximum bei einer Außentemperatur von 18–22° C mit einer dauerhaften Steigerung auf 200–300 Kcal/h [5]. Die Steuerung besteht aus einer peripheren Kältestimulation und einer zentralen Wärmeinhibition [5]. Beim Menschen scheint die zentrale Steuerung, wie bei vielen größeren Säugetieren, den Vorrang über die periphere Steuerung mit einem Faktor von 3 bis 7 zu haben [11]. Die maximale Stoffwechselreaktion kann bis auf 16.000 Kcal/24 h durch heftiges Muskelzittern ansteigen. Wenn ein Stimulus wie z. B. Wasser mit 12° C so stark ist, daß er diese Reaktion auslöst, kann trotzdem ein Absinken der Körpertemperatur nicht mehr vermieden werden. Die maximale dauerhafte Reaktion entspricht einer Steigerung auf 6000–7000 Kcal/24 h [5]. Gleichzeitig mit dem Anstieg der Stoffwechselrate kommt es zu einer peripheren Vasokonstriktion. In den konstringierten Gebieten ist einerseits der Wärmeverlust vermindert, andererseits dienen diese als Wärmedämmung für den Kern. Unterschiedlichen Strategien der Natur haben sich bei der Adaptation kälteexponierter Bevölkerungsgruppen feststellen lassen. Während bei Australischen Buschmännern kein Anstieg der metabolischen Wärmeproduktion während der kalten Nächte gefunden wurde, obwohl die mittlere Körpertemperatur kontinuierlich abfiel und eine ausgeprägte Vasokonstriktion auftrat, fand man bei Eskimos und weißen Nordamerikanern einen adäquaten Anstieg der metabolischen Wärmeproduktion bei Abfall der mittleren Körpertemperatur [23, 24]. Die Eskimos wiesen zusätzlich eine deutlich geringere periphere Vasokonstriktion auf. Nach einer Expedition zum Nordpol weisen Mitteleuropäer die typische metabolische Antwort auf Kälteexposition auf. Allerdings setzt diese bei niedrigeren zentralen Temperaturen ein und die Peripherie bleibt offener mit entsprechend höheren Hauttemperaturen [7].

Wenn die Körpertemperatur trotz Gegenregulation zu sinken beginnt, treten bei 34° C Störungen der Aufmerksamkeit ein, bei 30° C beginnt die maximale Stoffwechselrate selbst zu sinken, bei 27° C sistiert die spontane Motorik außer jene der ventilatorischen Muskulatur, welche bei 25° C zum Stillstand kommt. Das Myokard ist um 30–32° C sehr vulnerabel und reagiert häufig mit Kammerflimmern.

Umgebungstemperatur und Stoffwechsel beim kritisch Kranken

Die metabolische Gegenregulation bei Kälteexposition ist beim relaxierten Patienten in Narkose deutlich vermindert. Bei diesen Patienten wird bei intensiver Oberflächenkühlung ein Abfall der Stoffwechselrate um 9 % pro ° C erreicht [31]. Die Schwelle für die vaskuläre Gegenregulation ist in N_2O/Opiatnarkose deutlich auf 34,2° C abgesenkt [50]. Die therapeutische Senkung der Stoffwechselrate wurde auch wiederholt für Intensivpatienten vorgeschlagen etwa im ARDS [59], bei erhöhtem Hirndruck [51], in der Schwangerschaft oder bei Kreislaufinsuffizienz. Diese Vorgangsweise bleibt umstritten [52], da bei nicht sedierten und nicht relaxierten Patienten eine deutliche metabolische Gegenregulation stattfinden kann [57] und z. B. bei Sepsis Hypothermie mit einer schlechteren Prognose verbunden ist [16].

Diese metabolische Gegenregulation auf Kälte sollte vermieden werden, da sie zumeist mit einem erhöhten Katabolismus vergesellschaftet ist. Dieser Effekt ist bei Verbrannten [4] und Neugeborenen [28] schon lange gesichert, wurde neuerdings aber auch für alle anderen Gruppen von Intensivpatienten postuliert [45]. Der erhöhte Katabolismus wurde mit einer erhöhten Ausschüttung von Cortisol in Zusammenhang gebracht, jedoch sind viele Fragen [37] noch offen, da nicht nur die Umgebungstemperatur sondern auch die Konstruktion des Bettes unterschiedlich waren.

Außer den metabolischen Nebenwirkungen einer Hypothermie wird auch die Sauerstoffverfügbarkeit beeinträchtigt, da die Fähigkeit, Sauerstoff zu extrahieren bei Hypothermie schlechter ist und daher ein früheres Einsetzen der Abhängigkeit des Sauerstoffverbrauchs vom Sauerstofftransport [47] manifest wird.

Hypothermie und Wiedererwärmung

Hypothermie mit Temperaturen unter 32° C begegnet dem Arzt in zweierlei Situationen. Einerseits kommt es zur akzidentellen Form durch Kälteexposition bei Bewußtlosigkeit, neurologischer Erkrankung oder Unfällen (Sturz ins Wasser oder Lawinen), andererseits kommt es zur therapeutischen Form im Rahmen von Herz und Gefäßoperationen mit extrakorporaler Zirkulation. Theoretisch würde die Stoffwechselrate um 7 %– 10 %/° C abfallen. Sowohl bei herzchirurgischen Eingriffen [42], wie bei der Wiedererwärmung neurologischer Patienten [6] lagen die Werte mit 4,5–5,3 %/° C deutlich niedriger. Das Ausmaß der Stoffwechselreduktion war stark unterschiedlich zwischen den Individuen und auch bei Temperaturen unter 20° C findet noch kein vollständiger metabolischer Stillstand statt.

Bei allen therapeutischen Verfahren sind folgende Richtlinien zu beachten:

1. eine rasche Abkühlung, die nach Erreichen des gewünschten Temperaturniveaus auch zeitlich so lange fortgeführt werden sollte bis eine homogene Kühlung vorliegt.

2. eine langsame Wiedererwärmung, wobei der Temperaturgradient zwischen zentralen Geweben und Blut 8–10° C nicht überschreiten sollte.

Bei der postoperativen Wiedererwärmung einer häufig beobachteten milden Hypothermie mit Temperaturen um 35° C bestehen zwei Möglichkeiten die metabolische Stimulation zu unterdrücken. Erstens kann das Muskelzittern durch Muskelrelaxation unterdrückt werden [43]. Dabei war in der relaxierten Gruppe einer Untersuchung, sowohl der Sauerstoffverbrauch geringer (–3,6 %) und damit die metabolische Wärmeproduktion geringer (–39 %) als auch der Wärmeverlust geringer (–50 %). Die paradoxe Beobachtung, daß die weniger vasokonstringierten

Patienten einen geringeren Wärmeverlust hatten, wurde dadurch erklärt, daß beim Muskelzittern relativ viel Wärme lokal verloren geht. Die Berechnung der Wärmeproduktion (WP) erfolgte aus dem Sauerstoffverbrauch (WP = $V'O_2$ × 4,94/Erwärmungszeit). Die Änderung des Wärmegehalts (delta BHC = 0,83 × Körpergewicht × (T1-T2)/Erwärmungszeit) des Körpers wurde aus der Temperaturänderung errechnet. Zweitens kann die metabolische Stimulation durch die Gabe von Opiaten ebenfalls in einer Größenordnung von 30 % vermindert werden [25, 44, 48]. Diese pharmakologischen Möglichkeiten der Stoffwechselökonomie müssen bei kardiorespiratorisch gefährdeten Patienten regelmäßig zum Einsatz kommen.

Fieber und Hyperthermie und Stoffwechsel

Fieber wird als eine Erhöhung der Körpertemperatur mit Verstellung der zentralen thermoregulatorischen Zielgröße („setpoint") definiert. Fieber wurde schon seit der Antike, als Krankheitssymptom gewertet. Hippokrates betrachtete Fieber als Trennung des „Kalten" und „Warmen" im Körper. Du Bois [18] untersuchte fiebernde Patienten gleichzeitig mittels direkter und indirekter Kalorimetrie während fieberhafter Erkrankungen wie Tuberkulose, Erysipel, Typhus, Arthritis etc. Er kam zum Schluß, daß die metabolische Wärmeproduktion (Stoffwechsel) um 13 %/° C ansteigt. Er gibt an, daß dieser Wert um 10–20 % erhöht werden muß, wenn ein starker Eiweißkatabolismus mit der Erkrankung verbunden ist oder wenn ausgiebig mit Eiweiß ernährt wird. Auf den Originalabbildungen von einzelnen Patienten läßt sich ganz klar ersehen, daß der größte Energieumsatz während des Anfieberns stattfindet und daß die Körpertemperatur noch lange, nachdem der Energieumsatz wieder abgefallen ist, erhöht bleibt. Während des Anfieberns kommt es auch zu einer veränderten Wärmeverteilung im Organismus aufgrund der Vasomotion, so daß bei anderen Untersuchungen [14] auch keine Beziehung zwischen Temperaturänderung und Änderung des Energieumsatzes gefunden wurde. Daher kann ein Anstieg der Kerntemperatur auch ein Zeichen von zirkulatorischer Zentralisation (Schock) sein und nicht von erhöhtem Energieumsatz.

Nicht definitiv geklärt ist die Annahme einer günstigen Wirkung von Fieber auf den Krankheitsverlauf [34, 19]. Allerdings scheint die Prognose von Patienten, die keine adäquate fieberhafte Reaktion bei Infekten erreichen, doch deutlich schlechter zu sein als bei Patienten mit Fieber. Bis zur definitiven Klärung sollte der Spontanverlauf der Körpertemperatur, solange sie unter 39,5–40° C gemessen wird oder der Patient nicht stark gestreßt ist, unbeeinflußt bleiben.

Häufig stellt sich bei kritisch Kranken die Frage nach der richtigen Menge der Energiezufuhr. Eine häufig angewandte Formel, wie jene von Harris-Benedict [17] überschätzt den Energiebedarf um 15 % aufgrund neuerer Studien an Gesunden. Andere rezente Messungen [53] an 112 beatmeten Patienten lassen Werte errechnen (1450 Kcal/m^2/24 h), die um ca. 50 % über jenen von Harris-Benedict (830 Kcal/m^2/24 h), Dubois (950 Kcal/m^{2y}/24 h), Brandi (1015 Kcal/m^2/24 h) oder Takala (950–1050 Kcal/m^2/24 h) liegen. Nachdem die Körpertemperatur der untersuchten Patienten in einem engen Bereich knapp über 37° C lag und die Energieumsätze so weit gestreut waren, scheint eine Vorhersage der Energieumsätze aufgrund der Körpertemperatur eines individuellen Patienten sehr schwierig. Ein praktikabler Zugang scheint die einfache Berechnung mit 25 Kcal/kg/24 h zu sein. Eine Korrektur mittels Streß- oder Aktivitätsfaktoren ist nur bei Verbrannten bzw. muskelaktiven Rekonvaleszenten zu empfehlen. Zusätzlich sollte mittels frühzeitiger Ernährung, die Möglichkeit, einen Hypermetabolismus stark zu dämpfen, genützt werden [15, 39].

Sepsis / Septischer Schock

Obwohl Fieber ein häufiges Symptom beim SIRS (systemic inflammatory reaction syndrome) darstellt, zeigten 10 % aller Patienten eine Hypothermie mit Temperaturen unter 35,5° C [16]. Die Prognose dieser Patienten war besonders schlecht. Bei Patienten nach Abdominalchirurgie im Multiorganversagen haben Patienten mit einem milden Hypermetabolismus (1140 Kcal/m^2/24 h bzw 31 Kcal/kg/24 h) das entspricht 41 % über den errechneten Werten nach Harris-Benedict eine deutlich bessere Prognose [21]. Bei den überlebenden Patienten war auch die

Körpertemperatur gering höher (0,6° C) als bei den nicht überlebenden. Kreymann [35] konnte zeigen, daß in der Sepsis der Energieumsatz um 55 %, im Sepsis Syndrom um 24 % und im Septischen Schock 2 % über den errechneten Werten nach Harris-Benedict lagen. Wenn man die Beziehung zur Körpertemperatur betrachtet, waren die höchsten Temperaturen bei den schockierten Patienten mit niedrigeren Energieumsätzen zu finden. Daher muß nicht nur bei postoperativen Patienten [14], sondern auch bei Patienten mit schweren Infektionen [35] Fieber nicht notwendigerweise einen erhöhten Energieumsatz bedeuten.

Spezifische dynamische Wirkung der Nährstoffe

Der nahrungsbedingte Energieumsatz bezeichnet jene Energie, die für die Absorption, den Umsatz und die Speicherung notwendig ist. Sie beträgt 6–8 % für Kohlenhydrate, 2–3 % für Fette und 30–40 % für Eiweiß [32]. Bei einer ausgewogenen Ernährung muß mit einem nahrungsbedingten zusätzlichen Energieumsatz von 10–15 % gerechnet werden. Im Normalfall kommt es nur zu minimalen Temperaturänderungen nach einer Mahlzeit. Bei unausgewogenen Ernährungsregimen (z. B. Glucose/Aminosäuren), die in großen Mengen [26] verabreicht werden, kann es zu einem deutlichen Anstieg des Energieumsatzes und der Körpertemperatur kommen [2]. Der thermogenetische Effekt der Aminosäurenzufuhr hängt sowohl von der Art der Aminosäuren [55], dem Zeitpunkt [27] wie der Phase der Erkrankung ab [49, 22]. Dabei reagieren septische und spontanatmende Patienten empfindlicher bei hoher Aminosäurenzufuhr.

Zusammenfassung

- Die Umgebungstemperatur auf der Intensivstation beeinflußt den Energieumsatz und ist nicht belanglos.

- Künstliche Kühlung kann eine deutliche Steigerung des Energieumsatzes bedingen.

- Erhöhte Körpertemperatur bedeutet erhöhten Energieumsatz oder Zentralisation mit oft erniedrigtem Energieumsatz.
- Die Vorhersage des individuellen Energieumsatzes ist nur beschränkt möglich. Im Zweifelsfall kann nur die (respiratorische) indirekte Kalorimetrie eine exakte Information liefern.
- Die Ernährung beeinflußt durch ihre Menge und ihre Zusammensetzung den Energieumsatz und die Körpertemperatur.

Literatur

1. Altman PL, Dittmer DS (eds) (1974) Biology data book, vol 3, 2nd edn. Fed Am Soc Exp Biol
2. Askanazi J, Rosenbaum SH, Michelsen CB, Elwyn DH, Hyman AI, Kinney JM (1980) Increased body temperature secondary to total parenteral nutrition. Crit Care Med 8: 736–737
3. Atwater WO, Benedict FG (1903) Experiments on the metabolism of matter and energy in the human body. 1900-1902. United States Department of Agriculture, Office of Experiment, Stations Bull No. 136. United States Government print office
4. Barr PO, Birke G, Liljedahl SO, Plantin LO (1968) Oxygen consumption and water loss during treatment of burns with warm dry air. Lancet i: 164–168
5. Benzinger TH (1969) Heat regulation: homeostasis of central temperature in man. Physiol Rev 49: 671–759
6. Biancolini CA, Del Bosco CG, Jorge MA, Poderoso JJ, Capdevila AA (1993) Active core rewarming in neurologic, hypothermic patients: effects on oxygen-realted variables. Crit Care Med 21: 1164–1168
7. Bittel JHM, Livecchi-Gonnot GH, Hanniquet AM, Poulain C, Etienne JL (1989) Thermal changes observed after J.L. Etienne's journey to the north pole. Is central nervous system temperature preserved in hypothermia? Eur J Appl Physiol 58: 646–651
8. Brandi LS, Grana M, Mazzanti T, Giunta F, Natali A, Ferrannini E (1992) Energy expenditure and gas exchange measurements in postoperative patients: thermodilution versus indirect calorimetry. Crit Care Med 20: 1273–1283
9. Bruder M, Dumont JC, Francois G (1991) Evolution of energy expenditure and nitrogen excretion in severe head-injured patients. Crit Care Med 19: 43–48
10. Bursztein S, Glaser P, Trichet B, Taitelman U, Nedey R (1980) Utilisation of protein, carbohydrate, and fat in fasting and postabsorptive subjects. Am J Clin Nutr 33: 998–1001

11. Cabanac M (1975) Temperature regulation. Ann Rev Physiol: 415–439
12. Cabanac M, Brinnel H (1987) The pathology of human temperature regulation: thermiatrics. Experientia 43: 19–27
13. Cabanac M, Brinnel H (1985) Blood flow in the emissary veins of the human head during hyperthermia. Eur J Appl Physiol 54: 172–176
14. Chiara O, Giomarelli PP, Bioagioli B, Rosi R, Gattinoni L (1987) Hypermetabolic response after hypothermic cardiopulmonary bypass. Crit Care Med 15: 995–1999
15. Chiarelli A, Enzi G, Casadei A, Baggio B, Valerio A, Mazzoleni F (1990) Very early nutrition supplementation in burned patients. Am J Clin Nutr 51: 1035–1039
16. Clemmer TP, Fisher CJ, Bone RC, Slotman GJ, Metz CA, Thomas FO (1992) Hypothermia in the sepsis syndrome and clinical outcome. Crit Care Med 20: 1395–1401
17. Daly JM, Heymsfield SB, Head CA, Harvey LP, Nixon TW, Katzeff H, Grossman GD (1985) Human energy requirements: overestimation by widely used prediction equation. Am J Clin Nutr 42: 1170–1174
18. Dubois EF (1921) The basal metabolism in fever. JAMA 5: 353–355
19. Duff GW (1986) Is fever beneficial to the host: a clinical perspective. Yale J Biol Med 59: 125–130
20. Erickson RS, Kirklin SK (1993) Comparison of ear-based, bladder, oral, and axillary methods for core temperature measurement. Crit Care Med 21: 1528–1534
21. Forsberg E, Soop, Thörne A (1991) Energy expenditure and outcome in patients with multiple organ failure following abdominal surgery. Intensive Care Med 17: 403–409
22. Giovannini I, Chiarla C, Boldrini G, Castiglioni GC, Castagneto M (1988) Calorimetric response to amino acid infusion in sepsis and critical illness. Crit Care Med 16: 667–670
23. Hammel HT, Elsner RW, Le Messurier DH, Andersen HT, Milan FA (1959) Thermal and metabolic responses of the Australian aborigine exposed to moderate cold in summer. J Appl Physiol 14: 605–615
24. Hart JS, Sabean HB, Hildes JA, Depocas F, Hammel HT, Andersen KL, Irving L, Foy G (1962) Thermal and metabolic responses of coastal Eskimos during a cold night. J Appl Physiol 17: 953–960
25. Hausmann D, Nadstawek J, Krajeski W (1991) O_2-Aufnahme in der Aufwachphase – Einfluß des Narkoseverfahrens und der postoperativen Pethidingabe. Anästhesist 40: 229–234
26. Henneberg S, Sjölin J, Stjernström H (1991) Over-feeding as a couse of fever in intensive care patients. Clin Nutr 10: 266–271
27. Hersio K, Takala J, Kari A, Huttunen H (1991) Changes in whole body and tissue oxygen consumption during recovery from hypothermia: effect of amino acid infusion. Crit Care Med 19: 503–508
28. Hey EN, O'Connell B. Oxygen consumption and heat balance in the cot-nursed baby. Arch Dis Childhood 45: 335–343

29. Hoar WS (1983) Temperature. In: Hoar WS (ed) General and comparative physiology, 3rd edn. Prentice Hall, New Jersey
30. Hunt LM (1969) An analytic formula to instantaneously determine total metabolic rate for the human system. J Appl Phys 5: 731–733
31. Hynson JM, Sessler D, Moayeri A, Mc Guire (1993) Absence of non-shivering. thermogenesis in anesthetized adult humans. Anesthesiology 79: 695–703
32. Iapichino G, Radrizzani D (1988) Metabolic support and energy supply for critically ill patients: a pathophysiological approach. Intensive Care World 2: 48–49
33. Kirvelä OA, Kanto JH (1991) Clinical and metabolic responses to different types of premedication. Anesth Analg 73: 49–53
34. Kluger MJ (1986) Is fever beneficial? Yale J Biol Med 59: 89–95
35. Kreymann G, Grosser S, Buggisch P, Gottschall C, Matthaei S, Greten H (1993) Oxygen consumption and resting metabolic rate in sepsis, sepsis syndrome, and septic shock. Crit Care Med 21: 1012–1019
36. Liggett SB, Renfro AD (1990) Energy exempeditures of mechanically ventilated nonsurgical patients. Chest 98: 682–686
37. Little RA (1990) Ambient temperature and postoperative catabolism. Intensive Care Med 16: 283–284
38. Mekjavic IB, Sundberg CJ, Linnarsson D (1991) Core temperature "null zone". J Appl Physiol 71: 1289–1295
39. Mochizuki H, Trocki O, Dominioni L, Brackett KA, Joffe SN, Alexander JW (1984) Mechanism of prevention of postburn hypermetabolism and catabolism by early enteral feeding. Ann Surg 200: 297–310
40. Pettenkofer M von (1862) Über die Respiration. Annal Chem [Suppl] 2: 1
41. Pflüger E (1878) Über die Wärme und Oxydation der lebendigen Materie. Arch Ges Physiol 18: 247
42. Prakash O, Jonson B, Bos E, Meij S, Hugenholtz PG, Hekman W (1978) Cardiorespiratory and metabolic effects of profound hypothermia. Crit Care Med 6: 340–346
43. Rodriguez JL, Weissman C, Damask MC, Askanazi J, Hyman AI, Kinney JM (1983) Physiologic requirements during rewarming: suppression of the shivering response. Crit Care Med 11: 490–497
44. Rodriguez J L, Weissman C, Damask MC, Askanazi J, Hyman AI, Kinney JM (1983) Morphine and postoperative rewarming in critically ill patients. Circulation 6: 1238–1246
45. Ryan DW, Clague MB (1990) Nitrogen sparing and the catabolic hormones in patients nursed at an elevated ambient temperature following major surgery. Intensive Care Med 16: 287–290
46. Ryan DW (1983) The influence of environmental temperature (32°C) on catabolism using the clinitron fluidised bed. Intensive Care Med 9: 279–281
47. Schumaker PT, Rowland J, Saltz S, Nelson DP, Wood LDH (1987) Effects of hyperthermia and hypothermia on oxygen extraction by tissues during hypovolemia. J Appl Physiol 63: 1246–1252

48. Semsroth M, Hiesmayr M (1990) Kontinuierliche Zufuhr von Morphium ist effektiver als Bolusgabe zur Analgosedierung im Kindesalter. Anästhesist 39: 552–556

49. Semsroth M (1985) Indirekte Kalorimetrie bei beatmeten polytraumatisierten Patienten. Infusionstherapie 12: 213–237

50. Sessler DI, Olofsson CI, Rubinstein EH (1988) The thermoregulatory threshold in humans during nitrous oxide-fentanyl anesthesia. Anesthesiology 69: 357–364

51. Steltzer H (1993) Abfall des Hirndrucks unter Hämofiltration mit leichter Hypothermie (persönliche Mitteilung)

52. Styrt B, Sugarman B (1990) Antipyresis and fever. Arch Intern Med 150: 1589–1597

53. Swinamer DL, Grace MG, Hamilton SM, Jones RL, Roberts P, King EG (1990) Preditive equation for assessing energy expenditure in mechanically ventilated critically ill patients. Crit Care Med 18: 657–661

54. Swinamer DL, Phang PT, Jones RL, Grace M, King EG (1988) Effect of routine administration of analgesia on energy expenditure in critically ill patients. Chest 92: 4–10

55. Takala J, Askanazi J, Weissman C, Lasala PA, Milic-Emili J, Elwyn DH, Kinney JM (1988) Changes in respiratory control induced by animo acid infusions. Crit Care Med 16: 465–469

56. Takala J, Keinänen O, Väisänen P, Kari A (1989) Measurement of gas exchange in intensive care: laboratory and clinical validation of a new device. Crit Care Med 17: 1041–1047

57. Wenzel C, Werner J (1988) Physical versus pharmacological counter measures. Eur J Appl Physiol 57: 81–88

58. Weir JB Ve D (1949) New methods for calculating the metabolic rate with special reference to protein metabolism. J Physiol 109: 1–9

59. Wetterberg T, Steen S (1992) Combined use of hypothermia and buffering in the treatment of critical respiratory failure. Acta Anaesthesiol Scand 36: 490–492

60. Williams RR, Fuenning CR (1991) Circulatory indirect calorimetry in the critically ill. JPEN 15: 509–512

61. Yousef (1987) Effects of climatic stresses on thermoregulatory processes in man. Experientia 43: 14–19

Korrespondenz: Dr. M. Hiesmayr, Abteilung für Herz-Thorax-Gefäßanästhesie und Intensivmedizin, AKH-Universität Wien, Währingergürtel 18–20, A-1090 Wien, Österreich

Metabolische Adaptation in der chronischen Hypoxie

B. Schneeweiß

Intensivstation, Klinik für Innere Medizin IV,
Universität Wien, Österreich

Einleitung

In hypoxietoleranten Spezies können im wesentlichen zwei
Strategien beobachtet werden, um unter chronisch hypoxischen
Bedingungen überleben zu können [1]: 1) Reduktion des Ener-
giebedarfs und somit des gesamten ATP-turnovers (= „metabolic
arrest") und 2) Verbesserung (= Erhöhung) der metabolischen
Effizienz. Die erstere Möglichkeit findet sich vor allem bei Tieren, die längere Zeit einer ausgeprägten Hypoxie bzw. auch An-
oxie ausgesetzt sind, ist aber dann nicht geeignet, wenn unter
chronischen Sauerstoffmangel weiter Arbeit geleistet werden
soll. Unter solchen Voraussetzungen wird hingegen bei aeroben
Organismen (wie auch beim Menschen) die zweite Möglichkeit,
eine Verbesserung der metabolischen Effizienz und Effizienz der
Zellarbeit realisiert.

Im Gegensatz zu den beschriebenen prinzipiellen Adap-
tionsmöglichkeiten an die chronische Hypoxie, werden unter
akut-hypoxischen Bedingungen eher anaerobe Stoffwechselwege
aktiviert, um die energetischen Voraussetzungen für das Aufrechterhalten der Zellintegrität zu erfüllen. Um allerdings den
Gesamtenergiebedarf durch die Aktivierung der nicht oxidativen
ATP-Produktion zu gewährleiten, muß bei der geringen ATP-
Ausbeute pro Mol Substrat der Substratdurchsatz deutlich gesteigert werden [2]. Diese Steigerung beträgt im Falle der anaeroben Glykolyse (dem quantitativ bedeutsamsten anaeroben
Stoffwechselweg beim Menschen) das 16-fache gegenüber der

oxidativen ATP-Produktion aus Glukose durch den Krebs-Zyklus und wird als *Pasteur-Effekt* bezeichent. Die durch den Pasteur-Effekt bedingte rasche Substratverarmung (Verbrauch der Glykogendepots) und somit Gefahr des energetischen Defizits sowie „Selbstvergiftung" durch die Endproduktakkumulation (im Falle der anaeroben Glykolyse Laktatproduktion und metabolische Azidose) machen diese metabolische Adapationsmölgichkeit für chronische hypoxische Zustände ungeeignet.

Das Laktatparadoxon

Werden Belastungsversuche bei nicht höhenakklimatisierten untrainierten und auch auf Kraft (Kurzzeitbelastung) trainierende Sportler durchgeführt, kommt es unter hypoxischen Bedingungen bei gleicher Belastungsstufe zu einer größeren Laktatproduktion als unter normoxischen Bedingungen [3, 4]. Dieses Phänomen findet durch den erwähnten Pasteur-Effekt eine Erklärung. Im Gegensatz dazu konnte Edwards bereits im Jahre 1936 zeigen, daß bei höhenakklimatisierten Personen (Andenbewohner) unter hypoxischen Bedingungen *weniger* Laktat produziert wird [5]. Diese Beobachtung wurde durch mehrere Arbeitsgruppen bestätigt und hat unter dem Namen *Laktatparadoxon* in die Literatur Eingang gefunden [6, 7].

Als Ursache für dieses Phänomen wurde eine verminderte anaerobe Glykolyserate gefunden [8]. Auf die dabei zugrunde liegenden Mechnismen soll im Folgenden näher eingegangen werden.

Veränderungen im Bereiche der anaeroben Glykolyse

Ob und welche Veränderungen im Bereiche der anaeroben Glykolyse unter chronisch hypoxischen (hypobare Hypoxie) Bedingungen auftreten, wurde von der Arbeitsgruppe um Housten untersucht [8, 9]. Diese Arbeiten wurden unter der Bezeichnung „*Operation Everst II*" publiziert und beschreiben unter anderem die metabolische Adaptation und Veränderungen im Sauerstoffverbrauch und -transport, wie sie unter einem simulierten (Unterdruckkammer) Aufstieg in eine Höhe die dem

Gipfel des Mt. Everest entspricht, auftreten. Die Untersuchungen wurden bei 760 Torr (= Meereshöhe), 380 Torr (= 6500 m) und 282 Torr (8100 m) durchgeführt. Die Akklimationszeit betrug bei 380 Torr 14 Tage, bei 282 Torr 21 Tage.

Dem Laktatparadoxon entsprechend, konnten mit sinkendem Umgebungsdruck unter einer maximalen Belastung niedrigere Laktatkonzentrationen gemessen werden [8] (Tabelle 1).

Tabelle 1

Luftdruck [Torr] [mMol/L]	Laktatkonzentration im Blut
760 Torr = Meereshöhe	$11,0 \pm 1,2$ (SE)
380 Torr = 6500 m	$8,1 \pm 0,8$
282 Torr = 8100 m	$5,2 \pm 0,7$

Der unter Belastung zu erwartende Anstieg der Muskelkonzentrationen der Metabolite der anaeroben Glykolyse Glukose-6-Phosphat (G-6-P), Fruktose-6-Phosphat (F-6-P), Glukose-1-Phosphat und Laktat war bei 282 Torr signifikant geringer ausgeprägt als bei 760 und 380 Torr. Diese Veränderungen im Bereiche der anaeroben Glykolyse waren nach Rückkehr auf 760 Torr innerhalb von 48 Stunden völlig reversibel. Die beschriebenen Veränderungen im Substratstoffwechsel wurden als *verminderte Aktivierung der anaeroben Glykolyse* und somit reduziertem Substratfluß von Glukose zu Pyruvat interprediert.

Die Mechanismen die für eine verminderte Laktatproduktion aus Pyruvat verantwortlich sind, können allerdings durch diese Beobachtungen allein noch nicht erklärt werden. In diesem Zusammenhang konnten P. Hochachka et al. [10] durch Enzymaktivitätsbestimmungen in Muskeln von Quechua Indianer ein deutlich erhöhtes Verhältnis der Pyruvatkinaseaktivität zur Laktatdehydrogenaseaktivität (PK/LDH Verältnis), bedingt durch eine verminderte LDH-Aktivität, finden. Ähnlich hohe PK/LDH Verhältnisse werden nur noch in der Flugmuskulatur des Kolibri gefunden [11]. Diese Muskulatur erbringt die höchsten bekannten aeroben Stoffwechselraten unter allen Vertebraten.

Neben der verminderten LDH-Aktivität konnte in der Muskulatur dieser Indianer eine hohe Malatdehydrogenease-Aktivität (MDH-Aktivität) gefunden werden. Hohe MDH-Aktivitäten konkurrieren mit LDH um das gemeinsame Substrat NADH im Rahmen des Malat-Asparat Shuttle (Reduktion mitochondraler NAD+durch im Cytosol im Rahmen der anaeroben Glykolyse produzierter NADH). D. h. auf Grund der verminderten LDH- und hohen MDH-Aktivität steht weniger NADH für die Laktatproduktion aus Pyruvat zur Verfügung.

Ähnliche Veränderungen der LDH- und MDH-Aktivitäten konnten bei auf Ausdauer trainierenden Sportlern gefunden werden [12].

Zusammenfassend können im Bereiche der anaeroben Glykolyse somit 3 Veränderungen gefunden werden, welche als Adaptionsmechanismen an eine chronische Hypoxie interprediert werden können und eine Erklärung für das bekannte Laktatparadoxon bieten:

1. verminderte anaeroben Glykolyserate
2. erhöhtes PK/LDH-Verhältnis
3. erhöhtes MDH/LDH-Verhältnis

Durch die besprochen metabolischen Veränderungen kann nun wohl die verminderte Laktatproduktion bei maximaler Belastung unter chronisch hypoxischen Bedingungen eine Erklärung finden, eine verminderte anaerobe Glykolyserate würde aber auch eine verminderte Energieproduktion bedeuten. Die metabolische Adaptation ist daher mit einer verminderten Leistungsfähigkeit verbunden: dem entsprechend konnte in der Studie „Operation Everest II" mit steigender Höhe (= vermindertem Sauerstoffpartialdruck) eine geringere maximale Leistungsfähigkeit gefunden werden [9]. Diese Veränderungen spiegeln somit das Phänomen des „metabolic arrest" als Mittel der biochemischen Adaptation, wie es von P. Hochachka beschrieben wurde, wider [1].

Andererseits konnte aber in der Studie „Operation Everest II" bei gleicher Arbeitsbelastung mit steigender Höhe ein geringerer Sauerstoffverbrauch gefunden werden. Diese Beobachtung wurde von Housten et al. [9] teilweise als gesteigerte mechanische Effizienz im Rahmen der fahrradergometrischen Untersuchung interprediert. Hochachka et al. konnten allerdings ein verbessertes energetisches „coupling" als Adaptation an die chronische Hypoxie finden [13].

Verbessertes energetisches Coupling als Adaption an die chronische Hypoxie

Inosin-Monophosphat (IMP), welches aus AMP in einer durch AMP-Deaminase katalysierten Reaktion gebildet wird und dessen Akkumulation in der Muskulatur in einem stöchiometrischen Verhältnis zur ATP-Verarmung steht, zeigte in der Studie „Operation Everest II" wohl bei 760 Torr einen signifikanten Anstieg, bei 380 Torr und 282 Torr konnte ein solcher allerdings nicht mehr festgestellt werden [8]. Wird das Verhältnis aus ATP-Verarmung (= IMP-Akkumulation) zu totalem ATP-turnover als Maß für die Imbalanz zwischen ATP-Produktion und ATP-Verbrauch, d. h. des „energy coupling" definiert [10], so kann der fehlende IMP-Anstieg in der chronischen Hypoxie als Hinweis für eine engere Koppelung zwischen Energiebedarf und Energieproduktion interprediert werden.

In einer Studie von Matheson et al. [13], welche an höhenadaptierten Andenbewohnern, nicht höhenadaptierten Sportlern welche auf Ausdauer bzw. auf Kurzzeitbelastung trainierten und an untrainierten Kontrollpersonen durchgeführt wurde, konnten folgende prozentuellen Werte für die Imbalanz der energetischen Koppelung in der Wadenmuskulatur gefunden werden (Tabelle 2).

Tabelle 2

	%Imbalanz der energetischen Koppelung
Höhenadaptierte Andenbewohner	0,24%
Sportler (Ausdauer)	0,29%
Sportler (Kurzzeitbelastung)	0,41%
Untrainierte Kontrollpersonen	0,80%

D. h. die ATPase-ATPsyntheseraten waren in der Wadenmuskulatur der Andenbewohner 3.3 mal besser aufeinander abgestimmt als bei untrainierten nicht höhenadaptierten Normalpersonen.

Wendet man das gleiche Konzept für der Berechnung der Imbalanz der energetischen Koppelung auf die Daten von Housten et al. aus der Studie „Operation Everest II" [8] an, so konnten folgende Daten an den verschiedenen Höhen aus den ge-

Tabelle 3

Luftdruck [Torr]	%Imbalanz der energetischen Koppelung
760 Torr = Meereshöhe	0,83%
380 Torr = 6500 m	0,31%
282 Torr = 8100 m	0,22%

messenen ATP-Umsatzraten und IMP-Konzentrationen berechnet werden [10] (Tabelle 3).

Wie schon in der Diskussion über die Veränderungen im Bereiche der anaeroben Glykolyse erwähnt, war die Laktatproduktion und somit die Glykolyserate bei niedrigeren Luftdrucken d. h. besserer energetischer Koppelung (= geringerer Imbalanz) vermindert (Tabelle 1).

Zusammenfassung

Im Rahmen der Adaptation an die chronische Hypoxie wird die Effizienz der aeroben ATP-Produktion durch Verbesserung der energetischen Koppelung zwischen ATP-Produktion und ATP-Verbrauchsrate gesteigert. Dadurch kann die Aktivität der anaeroben Glykolyse vermindert werden.

Durch Veränderung im Aktivitätsmuster verschiedener Enzyme der anaeroben Glykolyse (hohes PK/LDH- und MDH/LDH-Verhältnis) findet das seit vielen Jahren bekannte Laktatparadoxon eine Erklärung.

Die beschriebenen Veränderungen im Intermediärstoffwechsel verhindern in der chronischen Hypoxie die Substratverarmung und Endproduktakkumulation (Laktatakkumulation) mit den möglichen Folgen und ungünstigen Auswirkungen einer metabolischen Azidose oder eventuell auch des Zelltodes.

Literatur

1. Hochachka PW, Guppy M (1987) Metabolic arrest and the control of time. Harvard University Press, Cambridge Ma London, pp 10–35

2. Hochachka PW, Guppy M (1987) Metabolic arrest and the control of time. Harvard University Press, Cambridge Ma London, pp 187–201

3. Knuttgen HG, Saltin B (1973) Oxygen uptake, muscle high energy phosphates and laactate in exercise under acute hypoxic conditions in man. Acta Physiol Scand 87: 368–376

4. Kobayashi K, Nelly JR (1979) Control of maximum rates of glycolysis in rat cardiac muscle. Circ Res 44: 166-175

5. Edwards HT (1936) Lactic acid in rest and work at high altitude. Am J Physiol 116: 367–375

6. Cerretelli PA, Veigsteinas A, Marconi C (1982) Anaerobic metabolism at high altitude. In: Brendal W, Zink RA (eds) High altitude physiology and medicine. Springer, New York, pp 94–162

7. West JB (1986) Lactate during exercise at extreme altitude. Fed Proc 45: 2953–2957

8. Green HJ, Sutton J, Young P, Cymerman A, Houston CS (1989) Operation Everest II: muscle energetics during maximal exhaustive exercise. J Appl Physiol 66(1): 142–150

9. Sutton JR, Reeves JT, Wagner PD, Groves BM, Cymerman A, Malconian MK, Rock PB, Young PM, Walter SD, Houston CS (1988) Operation Everst II: Exygen transport during exercise at extreme simulated altitude. J Appl Physiol 64(4): 1309–1321

10. Hochachka P W (1993) Adaptability of metabolic efficiencies under chronic hypoxia in man. In: Hochachka PW, Lutz PL, Sick T, Rosenthal M, van den Thillart G (eds) Surviving hypoxia. Mechanisms of control and adaptation. CRC Press, Boca Raton Ann Arbor London Tokyo, pp 127–135

11. Hochachka PW, Stanley C, McKenzie DC, Villena A, Monge C (1992) Enzyme mechanisms for pyruvate-to lactate flux attenuation: a study of Sherpas, Quechuas, and hummingbirds. Int J Sports Med 13: 119–126

12. Burke ER, Cerney B, Costill D, Fink W (1977) Characteristics of skeletal muscle in competitive cyclists. Med Sci Sports 9: 109–116

13. Matheson GO, Allen PS, Ellinger DC, Hanstock CC, Gheorghin D, McKenzie DC, Stanley C, Parkhouse WS, Hochachka PW (1991) Skeletal muscle metabolism and work capacity: a 31P-NMR study of Andean natives and lowlanders. J Appl Physiol 70: 1963–1971

Korrespondenz: Dr. B. Schneeweiß, Intensivstation 13 H1, Klinik für Innere Medizin IV, Universität Wien, Währinger Gürtel 18–20, A-1090 Wien, Österreich

Metabolismus bei Sepsis – Pathophysiologie

K. Ratheiser

Intensivstation, Klinik für Innere Medizin IV,
Universität Wien, Österreich

In der Folge von Traumen, Sepsis oder Operationen ereignen
sich vorhersagbare und gut erkennbare physiologische und metabolische Veränderungen, die sowohl den Glukose- wie auch
den Fett- und Eiweißstoffwechsel betreffen: erhöhter Grundum-
satz, Eiweißabbau, negative Stickstoffbilanz, Insulinresistenz,
erhöhte Insulinsekretion, gesteigerte Lipolyse und Streßhyperglykämie. Diese Veränderungen können in zwei unterschiedliche Perioden eingeteilt werden, nämlich in die (a) hy-
podyname Phase (*„ebb-phase"*), die unmittelbar nach Erkran-
kungsbeginn einsetzt, nur kurz andauert und durch den Abfall
von Blutdruck, Herzzeitvolumen und Sauerstoffverbrauch gekennzeichnet ist und die (b) hyperdyname Phase (*„flow-phase"*),
die mit einem „Hypermetabolismus" einhergeht, mit erhöhtem
„Cardiac output", mit negativer Stickstoffbilanz und Hyperglykämie.

Kohlenhydratstoffwechsel

In der initialen *„ebb-phase"* ist die Serumglukosekonzentration
erhöht, die basale endogene Glukoseproduktion ist noch normal
(1,2–2 mg/kg/min) bei reduzierter peripherer Insulinkonzen-
tration und erhöhtem Serumlaktat. In der *„flow-phase"* ändert
sich dieses Profil: während beim Gesunden ein erhöhter peripherer Glukosespiegel die hepatische Glukoseproduktion
hemmt, liegt bei der Sepsis wie auch bei Traumen oder Ver-

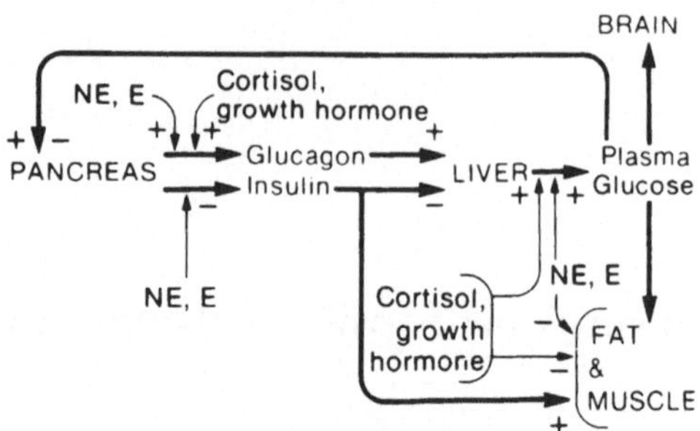

Abb. 1. Hormonprofil bei „Streßhyperglykämie": Die Glukosehomöostase wird vom endokrinen Pankreas, der Leber und den insulin-sensitiven Geweben geregelt. Das Gehirn ist in seiner Glukoseaufnahme nur von der Serumglukosekonzentration und von der cerebralen Durchblutung abhängig. Die Streßhormone Adrenalin (E; Epinephrin) und Noradrenalin (NE) haben als Inhibitoren der glukoseinduzierten Insulinsekretion eine zentrale Bedeutung

brennungen eine Resistenz der Leber gegenüber *Glukose* und *Insulin* vor. Zusätzlich zur fehlenden Hemmwirkung von Glukose und Insulin spielt das *Glukagon* eine Schlüsselrolle bei der Stimulation der hepatischen Glukoseproduktion [1]. Einen weiteren Beitrag zur „Streßhyperglykämie" liefert die hochgradige *Einschränkung der Glukoseaufnahme* in die peripheren (insulin-sensitiven) Gewebe, insbesondere die Muskulatur und das Fettgewebe, die sehr wahrscheinlich durch eine intrazelluläre Störung im Glukosemetabolismus („Postrezeptor-Defekt") bedingt ist [2]. Durch sympathische Aktivität wird die Lipolyse induziert und *Freie Fettsäuren (FFA)* werden freigesetzt, die die intrazelluläre Glukoseverwertung kompetitiv hemmen und damit einen wesentlichen Mechanismus für die Glukoseintoleranz darstellen. Auch ein erhöhter Insulin-Turnover trägt zur Insulinresistenz im Rahmen der Sepsis bei [3, 4]. „*Insulinresistenz*" ist jedoch nicht mit einem absoluten Glukose-Aufnahmestop in die insulinabhängigen Gewebe gleichzusetzen. Eine Steigerung der Glukoseaufnahme durch Insulininfusion ist bei Gesunden bis 15 mg/kg/min möglich, bei schwerer Streßexposition wie eben Trauma, Verbrennung oder Sepsis ist das Plateau der Glukoseaufnahme bereits bei 9 mg/kg/min erreicht, eine adäquate Zunahme der *Glukoseoxidation* ist aber nur bis zu einer Rate von 6 mg/kg/min gegeben. Jenseits dieser Grenze korrelieren Glukoseaufnahme in die Peripherie (Muskel-, Fettgewebe) und Glukoseoxidaton nicht mehr [2]. Es ist aber darauf hinzuweisen, daß es – in selteneren Fällen – im Rahmen einer schweren Sepsis auch zu einer Hypoglykämie kommen kann, nämlich dann, wenn das Endotoxin oder die sogenannten „Endotoxin-ähnlichen Substanzen" aus den Leukozyten die hepatische Glukoseproduktion direkt hemmen [5]. Somit kann bei einer Sepsis sowohl eine Hyperglykämie wie auch eine Hypoglykämie vorliegen.

Fettstoffwechsel

Fett stellt das größte Reservoir gespeicherter Energie dar. Bei Gesunden ist die FFA-Konzentration sehr eng korreliert mit der *FFA-Turnover-Rate* („rate of appearance" = endogene FFA-Freisetzungsrate) und deren Oxidation. Bei der Sepsis wie auch bei prolongiertem Fasten und nach Polytraumen wird das Fett zunehmend zum Hauptsubstrat für die Energiegewinnung. Freie Fettsäuren werden in einem Maß freigesetzt, das weit über dem Bedarf eines gesunden Organismus liegt und unabhängig vom jeweiligen FFA-Plasmaspiegel ist die FFA- und Glycerol-Turnoverrate höher als bei Normalpersonen [6]. Für die Aufnahme von Triglyzeriden ist die *Lipoprotein-Lipase (LPL)* verantwortlich. Dieses Enzym ist an das Kapillarendothel gebunden und in seiner Aktivität bei septischen Patienten erhöht [7]. Für das besondere Phänomen, daß die LPL-Aktivität bei Sepsispatienten im Muskelgewebe deutlich höher ist als im Fettgewebe kommt das *„Cachektin"* als Mediator in Frage, dessen Aufgabe es ganz offensichtlich ist, Fett vom Fettgewebe zu mobilisieren und dem Muskelgewebe als verwertbaren Nahrungsstoff zur Verfügung zu stellen.

Eiweißstoffwechsel

Zum klassischen metabolischen Befund bei Sepsis gehört der Eiweißabbau und die negative Stickstoffbilanz, wobei der Stickstoffverlust bis zu 30 Gramm pro Tag betragen kann. Der Abbau von Muskelproteinen führt zu vermehrtem Angebot von Präkursoren für die Glukoneogenese in der Leber. Zudem werden

für die Synthese von Akutphasenproteinen und Leukozyten
große Mengen an Aminosäuren und Glukose benötigt. Bei der
Sepsis erscheint die Eiweißspeicherung im Muskel jenen Substanzen gegenüber resistent zu sein, welche ansonsten den
Proteinabbau regulieren wie Insulin, Leucin oder die alpha-Ke-
toisokapronsäure. Die insulinmediierte Aminosäureaufnahme in
die Zellen (besonders der Muskulatur) ist gehemmt [8].

Proteinstoffwechsel und Leber

Vom teleologischen Standpunkt ist der Eiweißstoffwechsel bei
der Sepsis dahingehend verschoben, daß ein verminderter Aminosäure „uptake" in die Muskulatur dazu „gedacht ist", ein ver-
mehrtes Aminosäureangebot an die Leber zu liefern. Die hepatische Aminosäureaufnahme ist bei Streßzuständen gesteigert
und hier wiederum besonders bei Patienten mit schweren Infekten. Pearl und Mitarbeiter fanden eine Korrelation zwischen
dem „Outcome" bei Sepsis und der viszeralen Aminosäure-Auf-
nahme, die von diesen Autoren als „Zentrale Aminosäure-
Plasma-Clearance-Rate" bezeichnet wurde [9]. Bei jener Gruppe
an Sepsispatienten, die letztlich nicht überlebten, war diese
Clearancerate signifikant niedriger als bei jenen Patienten, die die
Sepsis überlebten.

Endokrine Mediatoren

Sowohl endokrine als auch zelluläre Mediatoren sind für die
komplette Manifestation der Sepsis im menschlichen Organismus
verantwortlich. Cortisol, Glukagon und Adrenalin induzieren
eine Zunahme des Grundumsatzes („Hypermetabolic state"), der
negativen Stickstoff- und Kaliumbilanz, der Glukose-Intoleranz,
der Hyperinsulinämie, der Insulinresistenz und der Natriumretention. Cortisol bewirkt darüberhinaus eine Zunahme der peripheren Freisetzung von Alanin und Glutamin aus dem Muskelgewebe und steigert auch die hepatische Glukoneogenese. Das
Glukagon hat sehr starke glykogenolytische und gluconeo-
genetische Auswirkungen auf die Leber. Eine Hyper-
glukagonämie vermehrt auch die Glutaminaufnahme in die Hepatozyten und in die Darmepithelzellen [10]. Das Wachstums-

hormon (GH) ist in der „flow-phase" der Sepsis erhöht. Der stickstoffsparende Effekt von GH wurde als Folge oder Begleiterscheinung einer vermehrten peripheren Fettoxidation identifiziert [11]. Auch das Schilddrüsenhormon Thyroxin, dessen Plasmaspiegel bei der Sepsis vermindert ist, könnte als endokriner Mediator wirken, da es im Tiermodell den Eiweißabbau hemmt und die Eiweißspeicher im Muskel wieder auffüllt [12].

Zelluläre Mediatorsysteme

– *Interleukin-1 (IL-1)* ist eine von aktivierten menschlichen Makrophagen abgeleitete Substanz, die den Muskeleiweißabbau „in vitro" vermehren kann und die hepatische Proteinsythese „in vivo" zu erhöhen vermag.

– *Proteolysis-inducing factor (PIF):* wurde von Clowes et al. definiert und hat dieselben Eigenschaften wie IL-1 [13]. Die adäquate Antwort auf den Mediator „PIF" wäre, die Freisetzung von Aminosäuren aus dem Organismus zu fördern (Eiweißabbau), damit diese für die Synthese von Antikörpern und anderen immunkompetenten Proteine zur Verfügung stehen. Sepsispatienten deren Aminosäure-Plasma-Clearancerate einen bestimmten Minimalwert unterschreitet, weisen eine höhere Mortalitätsrate auf [13]. Bei der Sepsis kommt es zu einer deutlichen Reduktion des Aminosäure-„uptakes" ins Muskelgewebe während das Pool an essentiellen Aminosäuren vergrößert ist. Dieser Effekt der Aminosäureaufnahme-Hemmung ins Muskelgewebe, der zu vermehrtem Aminosäureangebot an die Leber führt, ist einer zirkulierenden Substanz mit dem Molekulargewicht von etwa 30.000 Dalton zuzuschreiben [14]. Zudem zeigen in vitro Studien, daß die *Monokine* ebenso einen Effekt auf die hepatische Proteinsynthese haben könnten [15]. Die Monozyten im peripheren Blut sowie das retikuloendotheliale System in der Leber und Milz induzieren sowohl die Bildung von Interleukin 1 (IL-1) wie auch des Cachektin/Tumor Necrosis Faktors (TNF) [19]. Die TNF-Aktivität löst eine Kaskade von biologischen Effekten aus, die zur letalen Endotoxinämie führen können. Diese Effekte setzen einen intakten adrenalen Kortex voraus und sind größtenteils durch Insulin reversibel. Angesichts der vorhin erwähnten erhöhten Insulinclearance bei der Sepsis können hier höhere Insulin-Infusionsraten erforderlich sein. In einer weiteren Studie wurde das *Bradykinin* untersucht, das bei niedriger Infusionsrate die endogene Glukosefreisetzung und hier wiederum vor allem die Glukoseneogenese aus Aminosäuren unterdrücken kann [16]. Bradykinin kann also als Stickstoff-sparender Mediator wirken.

Andere Monokine wie die „macrophage insulin-like activity" (MILA) stimulieren die Glukoseoxidation.

Mineralhaushalt bei Sepsis

Bei septischen Zuständen treten Verschiebungen im Haushalt von Magnesium, anorganischem Phosphat, Zink und Kalium vorwiegend im intrazellulären, weniger im extrazellulären Milieu auf. Dabei kommt es zu einem intrazellulären Mangel an Magnesium und Phosphat wobei letzterer die Zwerchfellkontraktilität beeinträchtigen kann. Im Rahmen von totaler parenteraler Ernährung (TPN) sind viele Fälle von Phosphatmangel beschrieben worden, wobei einige sogar letal verliefen. Tremor, Parästhesien, Schwäche, verebrale Krampfanfälle und Koma sind die Hauptsymptome.

Bei schweren Infektionserkrankungen kommt es zu einem exzessiven Zink-Verlust, der sich oft der Diagnostik aus dem Serum entzieht und der einen negativen Effekt auf die Energiegewinnung und die Immunabwehr mit sich bringt [17]. Daher lassen erhöhte gastrointestinale Elektrolytverluste, ein hypermetabolischer Status wie chronische Aminosäurezufuhr eine zusätzliche Zinkgabe als sinnvoll erscheinen.

Das Eisen scheint im Rahmen der Sepsis in der Leber zu akkumulieren, was ebenso zu einer Beeinträchtigung des Immunstatus führt. Auch ein Seleniummangel kann während der TPN entstehen wobei sowohl Muskelschmerzen wie auch eine sekundäre Kardiomyopathie bei Patienten mit Langzeit-TPN mit einem Seleniummangel in Verbindung gebracht wurden.

Energiehaushalt

Der Gehalt an energiereichem Phosphat im Muskelgewebe ist bei der Sepsis vermindert [18]. Dieser Abfall von ATP ist be-

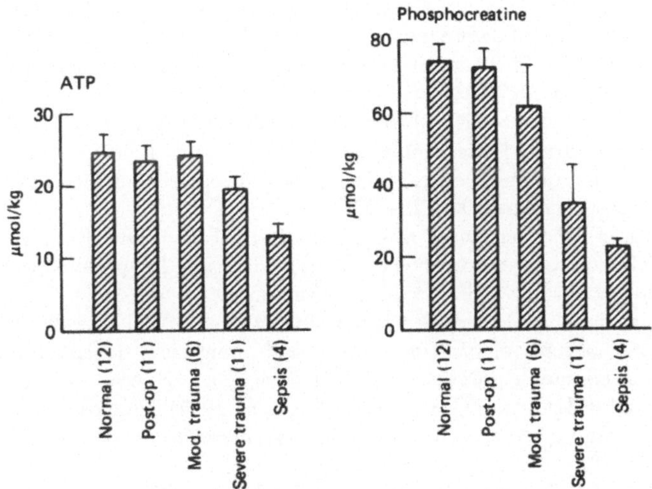

Abb. 2. Muskelenergiegehalt (ATP und Phosphokreatinspiegel; Mittelwert ± SD) in µg/kg bei Normalpersonen und Patienten nach operativen Eingriffen, Patienten mit mäßiggradigem oder schwerem Trauma sowie bei Patienten mit Sepsis [18]

gleitet von einem intrazellulären Kalium- und Magnesiummangel. Der Energiegehalt einer Zelle ist bestimmt durch die relativen Konzentrationen von Adenosinmono-, di- und triphosphat (AMP, ADP und ATP). Niedriger Energiegehalt wurde bei Patienten mit Schwersterkrankungen wie respiratorischem Versagen, Mangelernährung, Trauma oder Sepsis gefunden (Abb. 2).

Wenn dieser intrazelluläre ATP-Mangel exzessiv ist, dann ist auch bei aggressiver Ernährungstherapie der zelluläre Untergang unaufhaltsam, was letztlich zum *„sick cell syndrome"* und Tod führen kann.

Literatur

1. Jahoor F, Herndon DN, Wolfe RR (1986) The role of insulin and glucagon in the response of glucose and alanine kinetics in burn-injured patients. J Clin Invest 78: 807–814

2. Black PR, Brooks DC, Bessey PQ, et al (1982) Mechanisms of insulin resistance following injury. Ann Surg 196: 420–435

3. Dahn MS, Lange P, Mitchell RA, Lobdell K, Wilson RF (1987) Insulin production following injury and sepsis. J Trauma 27: 1031–1037
4. Wolfe RR (1987) Carbohydrate metabolism in the critically ill patient. Crit Care Clinics 3: 11–24
5. Miller SI, Wallace RJ, Musher DM, et al (1980) Am J Med 68: 649–654
6. Nordenstrom J, Carpentier YA, Askanazi J, et al (1983) Free fatty acid mobilisation and oxidation during total parenteral nutrition in trauma and sepsis. Ann Surg 198: 725–735
7. Robin AP, Greenwood MRC, Askanazi J, Elwyn DH, Kinney JM (1981) Influence of total parenteral nutrition on tissue lipoprotein lipase activity during chronic and acute illness. Ann Surg 194: 681–686
8. Hasselgren PO, Pedersen P, Sax HC, Warner BW, Fisher JE (1988) Current concepts of protein turnover and amino acid transport in liver and skeletal muscle during sepsis. Arch Surg 123: 992–999
9. Pearl RH, Clowes GHA, Hirsch EF, et al (1985) Prognosis and survival as determined by visceral amino acid clearance in severe trauma. J Trauma 25: 777–783
10. Geer RJ, Williams PE, Lairmore T, Abumrad NN (1987) Glucagon: an important stimulator of gut and hepatic glutamine metabolism. Surg Forum 37: 27–29
11. Suchner U, Rothkopf MM, Stanislaus G, et al (1990) Effects of growth hormone and total parenteral nutrition in patients with chronic obstructive pulmonary disease and malnutrition. Arch Intern Med 150: 1225–1230
12. Hasselgren PO, Chen AW, James JH, Sperling M, Warner BW, Fisher JE (1987) Studies on the possible role of thyroid hormone in altered muscle protein turnover in sepsis. Ann Surg 206: 18–24
13. Clowes GHA, Hirsch E, George GC, et al (1985) Survival from spesis: the significance of altered protein metabolism regulated by proteolysis inducing factor, the circulating cleavage product of interleukin-1. Ann Surg 202: 446–458
14. Hasselgren PO, James JH, Fisher JE (1985) Inhibited muscle amino acid uptake in sepsis. Ann Surg 203: 360–365
15. Le PT, Martensen RF (1984) In vitro induction of hepatocyte synthesis of the acute phase reactant mouse amyloid P-component by macrophages and IL-1. J Leuk Biol 35: 587–603
16. Sheldon GF (1988) Trauma and burns. Am Coll Surg Bull 73: 37–41
17. Chandra RK (1983) Nutrition immunity and infection: present knowledge and future directions. Lancet i: 688–691
18. Liaw KY, Askanazi J, Michelson CB, Kantrowitz LR, Fürst P, Kinney JM (1980) Effect of injury and Sepsis on high energy phosphates in muscle and red cells. J Trauma 20: 775–759
19. Nathan CF (1987) Secretory products of macrophages. J Clin Invest 79: 319–326

Korrespondenz: Dr. K. Ratheiser, Intensivstation, Klinik für Innere Medizin IV, Währingergürtel 18–20, A-1090 Wien, Österreich

Pathophysiologie der Azidose bei Sepsis

R. S. Hotchkiss

Department of Anesthesiology, Washington University School of Medicine,
St. Louis, MO, U.S.A.

Die Sepsis geht in der Regel mit einer Anzahl von metabolischen Störungen einher: Erhöhte Plasmalaktatkonzentration, metabolische Azidose, verstärkte Glykolyse und ein abnormer „transportabhängiger" Sauerstoffverbrauch. Es bestehen heute zwei Hypothesen zur Erklärung dieser Veränderungen:

a) Die zelluläre Hypoxie resultiert aus einer pathologisch veränderten Mikrozirkulation.

b) Es besteht eine primäre Störung im zellulären Energiestoffwechsel.

Tierexperimentelle Untersuchungen weisen darauf hin, daß kein bioenergetisches Versagen im septischen Gewebe besteht und daß die Zunahme der Laktatkonzentration nicht unbedingt auf eine zelluläre Hypoxie zurückzuführen ist. Die ausreichende zelluläre Oxygenation und Bioenergetik wurde durch in vivo Untersuchungen mit Hilfe der Nuklearmagnetresonanzspektroskopie und mikrofluorometrischen Enzymtechniken gefunden. Diese Untersuchungen weisen zusammen mit klinischen Untersuchungen darauf hin, daß keine der beiden Hypothesen ausreichend die pathologischen Veränderungen im Rahmen der Sepsis erklären kann.

1. Plasmalaktatkonzentration und Laktatazidose

1.1 Ätiologie der erhöhten Plasmalaktatkonzentration mit/ohne Azidose

a) Vermindertes effektives Blutvolumen mit konsekutiver zellulärer Hypoxie.

b) Gewebeischämie durch AV-, bzw. physiologische Shunts.

c) Eingeschränkte Aktivität der Pyruvatdehydrogenase. Die PDH war im Muskelgewebe (aber nicht Leber) septischer Ratten signifikant verringert [13]. Diese war durch Dichloroazetat reversibel [14]. Bei Patienten mit Verbrennungen und/oder Sepsis konnte dies jedoch nicht bestätigt werden [7].

d) Erhöhter Aminosäurenverfügbarkeit (durch erhöhten Eiweißabbau)

e) Verminderte Laktatclearance (Leberinsuffizienz, Niereninsuffizienz)

f) Verstärkte Erythrozytenproduktion: Das produzierte Laktat stammt hauptsächlich aus Muskel und Erythrozyten. Bei septischen Ratten konnte jedoch keine vermehrte Laktatproduktion durch Erythrozyten gefunden werden [4].

g) Erhöhte aerobe und nicht anaerobe Laktatproduktion: Durch verschiedene Stimuli kann die Glykolyse erhöht werden. Es entsteht hierbei vermehrt Pyruvat und Laktat (P/L Ratio bleibt gleich). Diese erhöhte aerobe Laktatbildung konnte tierexperimentell in septischen Geweben nachgewiesen werden [6].

1.2 Signifikanz der erhöhten Laktatkonzentration

a) Laktat ist weder ein sensitiver noch spezifischer Marker der zellulären Hypoxie weil: 1. Eine zelluläre Hypoxie kann ohne Laktaterhöhung einhergehen, weil die Aufnahme und die Verstoffwechselung des anaerob produzierten Laktats durch gut oxygenierte Zellen erfolgt. 2. Eine milde Laktaterhöhung kann eintreten ohne deswegen auf eine zelluläre Hypoxie hinweisen zu müssen.

b) Eine erhöhte Plasmalaktatkonzentration, die assoziiert ist mit einer Verminderung der Plasmabikarbonatkonzentration, vermindertem arteriellem pH-Wert, und/oder erhöhtem Kation/Anion Gap weist hin auf einen inadäquaten Flüssigkeitsersatz, verminderten Sauerstofftransport, und/oder lokale Gewebeischämie.

2. Untersuchungen der zellulären Hypoxie

2.1 Experimentelle Studien

a) Metabolische Parameter:
 - Zwischenprodukte der Glykolyse und des Krebszyklus, Laktat/Pyruvat Ratio
 - Bikarbonatkonzentration, Anion Gap
   $(Na^+ - (Cl^- + HCO^{3-}))$
b) ^{31}P Nuklearmagnetresonanzspektroskopie
 - pH_i
 - Phosphocreatine, ATP

Mit Hilfe dieser Methoden konnte im septischen Rattenmuskel keine Abnahme der Konzentration energiereicher Phosphate gefunden werden [6]. Obwohl tierexperimentell eine Abnahme des Muskelblutflusses um 33 % gefunden werden konnte, war der pH_i gleich wie in den Kontrolltieren [11]. Auch der Energiestoffwechsel des Gehirnes bei Ratten mit E.coli Sepsis war weitgehend unverändert, erst terminal kam es zu einem Abfall der energiereichen Phosphate und des pH_i [3]. Auch im Bereich des Herzmuskels konnten keine Veränderungen gefunden werden. Sowohl die Stoffwechselprodukte des Krebszyklus als auch die energiereichen Phosphate (hier liegen jedoch unterschiedliche Ergebnisse vor) waren nicht signifikant verändert gegenüber Kontrolltieren [5]. Gefunden wurde eine erhöhte Phosphocholinkonzentration, wahrscheinlich als Ausdruck einer erhöhten Membrandegradation, eine Abnahme der Alanin und Glutamatkonzentration.

Theoretisch wäre allerdings möglich, daß obwohl genügend Sauerstoff für die ATP Produktion vorhanden ist, andere Sauerstoff verbrauchende Prozesse, die in die Biosynthese oder Biodegradation involviert sind, beeinträchtigt sind.

2.2 *Klinische Studien*

a) 1. Abhängigkeit des VO2 vom DO2. Beim Gesunden steigt der Sauerstoffverbrauch bei Zunahme des Sauerstofftransportes bis zu einer gewissen Größe an, danach bleibt er konstant, unabhängig von einer weiteren Zunahme des Sauerstofftransportes. Im Gegensatz dazu wurde bei Patienten mit Sepsis eine weitere Zunahme des Sauerstoffverbrauches über einen weiten Bereich des Sauerstofftransportes der über den bei Gesunden hinausgeht beobachtet [10]. Diese transportabhängige Sauerstoffaufnahme wird als Sauerstoffmangel der Zelle angesehen und der inadäquate Transport als wichtiger Faktor für die Entstehung des Multiorganversagen diskutiert. In weiteren Studien wurde darauf hingewiesen, daß durch Verbesserung des Sauerstofftransportes auf supranormale Werte durch positiv inotrope Substanzen und Volumen, das Überleben verbessert werden kann [9]. Gegen diese Annahmen spricht, a) daß die transportabhängige Verbrauchssteigerung nicht typisch für Sepsis ist, sondern auch bei pulmonaler Hypertension, Schlafapnoe und Lebererkrankungen [8, 15] gefunden werden kann, ohne daß Zeichen einer Hypoxie sichtbar wären; b) bei Berechnung von DO2 und VO2 aus dem HZV besteht das Problem der mathematischen Kupplung, wird der VO2 mit einer anderen Methode bestimmt, so konnte bei ARDS-Patienten keine Abhängigkeit des VO2 vom DO2 mehr gefunden werden [1]; c) eine Zunahme des Blutflusses kann in einigen Organen zu einer Zunahme des Sauerstoffverbrauches führen, z. B. eine Zunahme des Herzminutenvolumen geht mit einer Zunahme des myokardialen VO2 einher.

a) 2. Metabolische Unterdrückung als protektiver Mechanismus.

b) Magen Mucosa pH-Bestimmung mit Hilfe der Tonometrie

c) Metabolische Studien:

Laktatextraktion: Eine erhöhte Laktatproduktion ist ein früher Indikator der zellulären Hypoxie. Bei Patienten mit Sepsis fand sich eine erhöhte myokardiale Laktataufnahme im Vergleich zu Patienten, bei denen eine Herzklappenoperation durchgeführt worden war [2], eine ischämisch/hypoxische Komponente scheint daher bei der myokardialen Funktionseinschränkung im Rahmen der Sepsis eher keine Rolle zu spielen. Die Laktatextraktion in der Leber war bei Patienten mit Verbrennung und Sepsis doppelt so hoch wie bei Gesunden [16]. D. h. auch im Bereich der Leber scheint keine Ischämie/Hypoxie als Sepsisfolge aufzutreten. In Untersuchungen am Muskel wurden erhöhte Laktat- und Pyruvatkonzentrationen gefunden [12], dies wurde jedoch nicht auf einen anaeroben Stoffwechsel zurückgeführt, daß die L/P Ratio gleich geblieben war und das Verhältnis der Verminderung der PCr-Konzentration zur Abnahme der ATP-Konzentration nicht typisch für die zelluläre Hypoxie war.

Literatur

1. Annat G, Viale JP, Percival C, Froment M, Motin J (1986) Oxygen delivery and uptake in the adult respiratory distress syndrome: lack of relationship when measured independently in patients with normal blood lactate concentrations. Am Rev Resp Dis 133: 999–1001

2. Dhainaut JF, Huyghebaert MF, Monsallier JF (1987) Coronary hemodynamics and myocardial metabolism of lactate, free fatty acids, glucose an ketones in patients with septic shock. Circulation 75: 533–541

3. Hochtkiss RS, Long RC, Hall JR (1989) An in vivo examination of rat brain during sepsis with ^{31}P-NMR spectroscopy. Am J Physiol 257: C1055–C1061

4. Hotchkiss RS, Song SK, Ling CS, Ackerman JJ, Karl IE (1990) Sepsis does not alter red blood cell glucose metabolism or Na$^+$ concentration: a ^{2}H-^{22}Na-NMR study. Am J Physiol 258: R21–R31

5. Hotchkiss RS, Song SK, Neil JJ (1991) Sepsis does not impair tricarboxylic acid cycle in the heart. Am J Physiol 260: C50–C57

6. Hotchkiss RS, Karl IE (1992) Reevalution of the role of cellular hypoxia and bionergetic failure in sepsis. JAMA 267: 1503–1510

7. Jahoor F, Shangraw RE, Miyoshi H, Wallfish H, Herndon DN, Wolfe RR (1989) Role of insulin and glucose oxidation in mediating the protein catabolism of burns and sepsis. Am J Physiol 257: E323–E331

8. Mohsenifar Z, Jasper AC, Koerner SK (1988) Relationship between oxygen uptake and oxygen delivery in patients with pulmonary hypertension. Am Rev Respir Dis 138: 69–73

9. Shoemaker WC, Appel PL, Kram HB (1988) Tissue oxygen debt as a determinant of lethal and nonlethal postoperative organ failure. Crit Care Med 16: 1117–1120

10. Shumacker PT, Samsel RW (1990) Oxygen supply and consumption in the adult respiratory distress syndrome. Clin Chest Med 11: 715–722

11. Song SK, Hotchkiss RS, Karl IE, Ackerman JJH (1993) Concurrent quantification of tissue metabolism and blood flow via ^{2}H/^{31}P NMR in

vivo. III. Alteration of muscle blood flow and metabolism during sepsis. Magn Reson Med (in press)

12. Tresadern JC, Threlfall CJ, Wilford K, Irving MH (1988) Muscle adenosine 5'triphosphate and creatine phosphate concentration in relation to nutritional status and sepsis in man. Clin Sci 75: 233–242

13. Vary TC, Siegel JH, Nakatani T, Sato T, Aoyama H (1986) Effect of sepsis on activity of pyruvate dehydrogenase complex in skeletal muscle and liver. Am J Physiol 250: E634–E640

14. Vary TC, Siegel JH, Fall BD, Morris JH (1988) Metabolic effects of partial reversal of pyruvate dehydrogenase activity by dichloroacetate in sepsis. Circ Shock 24: 3–18

15. Williams AJ, Mohsenifar Z (1989) Oxygen supply dependency in patients with obstructive sleep apnea and its reversal after therapy with nasal continuous positive airway pressure. Am Rev Resp Dis 140: 1308–1311

16. Wilmore DW, Goodwin CW, Pruitt BA (1980) Effect of injury and infection on visveral metabolism and circulation. Ann Surg 192: 491–504

Korrespondenz: R. S. Hotchkiss, M. D., Ass. Prof., Department of Anesthesiology, Washington University School of Medicine, 660 S Euclid Ave, Box 8054, St. Louis, MO 63110, U. S. A.

Thiaminmangel als Ursache der Laktazidose

C. Madl, A. Kranz, W. Druml und K. Lenz

Intensivstation, Klinik für Innere Medizin IV,
Universität Wien, Österreich

Thiamin (Vitamin B1) gehört zu den wasserlöslichen Vitaminen und besteht chemisch aus einem Pyrimidinring, der über eine Methylenbrücke mit dem aktiven Thiazolanteil verbunden ist. Im menschlichen Organismus sind ca. 25–30 mg Thiamin gespeichert, wobei ca. 80 % als Thiaminpyrophosphat, 10 % als Thiamintriphosphat und 10 % freies Thiamin vorliegen. Die biologisch aktive Form Thiaminpyrophosphat (= Cocarboxylase), wirkt als Coenzym bei wichtigen Reaktionen im Energiestoffwechsel [12]. Einerseits wirkt Thiaminpyrophosphat als Schlüsselenzym, in einem Multienzymkomplex mit der Pyruvatdehydrogenase, um das Endprodukt der Glykolyse Pyruvat in den Zitratzyklus einzuschleusen (Abb. 1). Zusätzlich wirkt es im Zitratzyklus als Coenzym bei der oxidativen Decarboxylierung von alpha-Ketoglutarat zu Succinyl-Co A und bei der Transketolasereaktion beim Pentosephosphatzyklus. Daraus geht hervor, daß es bei einem Thiamin-Mangel im Rahmen der gestörten Glykolyse zu einem Anfluten des Pyruvats mit konsekutiver erhöhter Umwandlung zu Laktat und zu einer beeinträchtigten Energiegewinnung im Zitratzyklus kommt (Abb. 1).

Da der menschliche Organismus nicht in der Lage ist Thiamin zu synthetisieren, erfolgt die Aufrechterhaltung des Thiaminhaushaltes ausschließlich über die Ernährung und über die Resorptionsfähigkeit des Gastrointestinaltraktes. Nach Empfehlung der American Medical Association Department of Foods

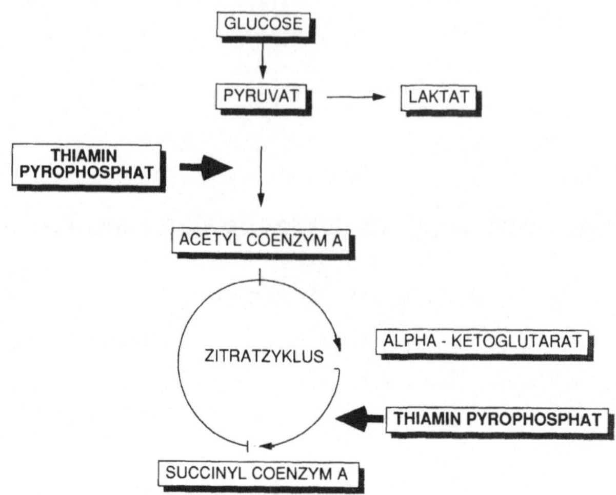

Abb. 1. Einfluß von Thiamin auf Stoffwechselreaktionen im Zitratzyklus

and Nutrition beträgt der tägliche Thiaminbedarf ca. 1–1,5 mg/ Tag. Da die Speicherfähigkeit des Organismus für Thiamin gering ist, liegt die biologische Halbwertszeit bei nur 10 bis 19 Tagen. Eine ausreichende und regelmäßige Zufuhr von Thiamin ist daher zur Vermeidung von Mangelzuständen notwendig.

Neben einer verminderten Thiaminzufuhr, führt vor allem ein erhöhter Thiaminverbrauch zu Thiaminmangelzuständen. Dazu zählen vor allem Erkrankungen mit großen Wundflächen, schwere Traumen, Infektionen, erhöhte Kohlenhydratzufuhr und Lebererkrankungen [9]. Aus diesem Grund erlangte der Thiaminhaushalt vor allem bei Intensivpatienten zunehmend an Interesse. Cruickshank et al. untersuchten bei 158 Intensivpatienten den Thiaminstatus [6]. Bereits zum Zeitpunkt der Aufnahme auf der Intensivstation bestand bei 20 % der Patienten der biochemische Nachweis eines Thiaminmangels. Bei diesen Patienten war die Mortalität mit 72 % deutlich höher im Vergleich zur Gesamtmortalität, die 50 % betrug. Außerdem war der Thiaminstatus bei Patienten die verstarben signifikant niedriger als bei jenen die überlebten. Die Inzidenz eines klinisch manifesten Thiaminmangels auf einer Intensivstation ist jedoch unbekannt zumal die Symptome dieser Hypovitaminose häufig

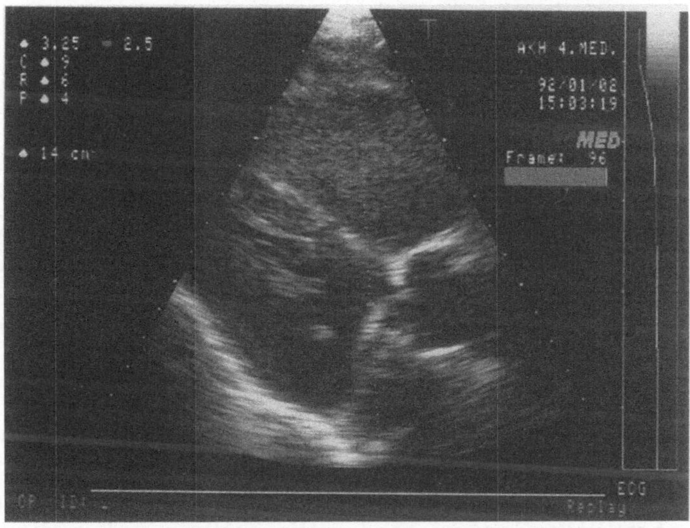

Abb. 2. Parasternaler Längsschnitt in transthorakaler Darstellung bei einer 66jährigen Patientin mit klinisch manifestem Thiaminmangel bei der Aufnahme auf die Intensivstation. Dabei zeigt sich eine isolierte Dilatation des rechten Ventrikels bei sonst unauffälligem altersentsprechendem Befund

unerkannt bleiben [11]. Einige Fallberichte belegen jedoch, daß Thiaminmangelzustände zu schweren klinischen Symptomen und sogar zum Tod führen können [2, 5, 7, 8, 10, 11]. Die klinischen Symptome des akuten Thiaminmangels sind charakterisiert durch eine schwere metabolische Azidose, Hyperlaktatämie, Senkung des peripheren Widerstandes mit Hypotonie, akutes Herzversagen und Natriumretention mit Ödembildung. Die Wernicke Enzephalopathie kann sich mit zerebralen Verwirrtheitszuständen bis zum Koma manifestieren. Fond et al. konnten außerdem exzessiv erhöhte Katecholaminspiegel in der akuten Phase nachweisen [7]. So war im Vergleich zu anderen Schockzuständen der Adrenalinspiegel 100 × höher. Zu Beginn der klinischen Manifestation scheint vorwiegend ein Rechtsherzversagen vorzuliegen ([8], Abb. 2). In weiterer Folge entwickelt sich jedoch ein biventrikuläres „high-output"-Versagen, dem ein Abfall des Herzminutenvolumens und der Auswurffraktion folgen kann. Dies dürfte auf eine mangelhafte

Energieversorgung des Myokards und auf eine durch die schwere metabolische Azidose hervorgerufene Hemmung der Katecholaminwirkung auf die Myokardzelle beruhen [9]. Diese kardialen Funktionsstörungen können jedoch durch eine ausreichende Thiaminsubstitution rückgängig gemacht werden. Gerade bei mangelhaft ernährten Patienten kann eine zusätzliche Infektion einen chronischen, asymptomischen Thiaminmangel in ein akutes klinisches Zustandsbild wandeln [8]. Vor allem eine unklare, therapierefraktäre Laktazidose und Hypotonie lassen den Verdacht auf einen Thiaminmangel zu.

Die Diagnostik eines Thiaminmangels kann durch biochemische Methoden erfolgen [1, 3, 4]. Die verläßlichste Methode ist die Bestimmung der Aktivität der Transketolase in den Erythrozyten. Die Erhöhung der Transketolaseaktivität nach Zusatz von Thiaminpyrophosphat wird als Thiaminpyrophosphat-Effekt gewertet und in Prozent angegeben. Eine Erhöhung des Aktivitätsgrades zwischen 15 und 25 % stellt einen milden Thiaminmangel, eine Erhöhung über 25 % einen schweren Mangel dar. Ein weiteres Kriterium für die Diagnose eines Thiaminmangels ist das Ausmaß der klinischen Reaktion auf Thiaminsupplementation. Eine rasche Besserung der vorher therapierefraktären metabolischen Azidose mit Abfall des Laktatspiegels und Besserung des Herzversagens nach ausreichender Thiaminzufuhr sind weitgehend beweisend für den Thiaminmangel.

Die Meinungen über die Dosierung der Therapie eines akuten Thiaminmangels wird jedoch noch kontrovers behandelt. Während Cruickshank et al. zu einer prophylaktischen Thiamingabe von 50 bis 250 mg bei jedem Patienten der auf der Intensivstation aufgenommen wird rät, schwanken die Therapieempfehlungen bei klinisch manifestem Thiaminmangel zwischen 100 und 500 mg/Tag [6, 9]). Eigene Beobachtungen mit einer Substitution von 600 mg Thiamin bei Patienten mit akutem Mangelzustand zeigten eine rasche Besserung der klinischen Symptomatik [8].

Bei unklarer, therapierefraktärer Laktazidose mit Hypotonie und Herzversagen muß ein Thiaminmangel in die Differentialdiagnose mit einbezogen werden. Eine Therapie mit hochdosierter Thiaminsubstitution scheint indiziert, zumal bei ausreichender Überwachung keine Nebenwirkungen zu erwarten sind. Das Ziel sollte jedoch sein, durch frühzeitige prophylaktische Thiaminsubstitution das Auftreten der Erkrankung zu vermeiden.

Literatur

1. Akbarian M, Dreyfus PM (1868) Blood transketolase activity in beriberi heart disease. A useful diagnostic index. J Am Med Assoc 203: 77–81
2. Attas M, Hanley HG, Stultz D, Jones MR, McAllister RG (1978) Fulminant beriberi heart disease with lactic acidosis: presentation of a case with evaluation of left ventricular function and review of pathophysiologic mechanisms. Circulation 58: 566–572
3. Bayoumi RA, Rosalki SB (1976) Evaluation of methods of coenzyme activation of erythrocyte enzymes for detection of deficiencies of vitamines B1, B2, and B6. Clin Chem 22: 327–331
4. Brin M, Tai M, Ostashever AS (1960) The effect of thiamine deficiency on the activity of erythrocyte hemolysate transketolase. J Nutr 71: 273–277
5. Campell CH (1984) The severe lacticacidosis of thiamine deficiency: acute pernicious or fulminanting beriberi. Lancet ii: 446–449
6. Cruickshank AM, Telfer ABM, Shenkin A (1988) Thiamine deficiency in the critically ill. Intensive Care Med 14: 384–387
7. Fond B, Richard C, Comoy E (1980) Two cases of shoshin beriberi with hemodynamic and plasma catecholamine data. Intensive Care Med 6: 193–198
8. Madl C, Kranz A, Liebisch B, Traindl O, Lenz K, Druml W (1993) Lactic acidosis in thiamine deficiency. Clin Nutr 12: 108–111
9. Neeser G, Eckhart J, Lichtwarck-Aschoff M, Wengert P, Adolph M (1989) Mangelsituation Vitamin B1. Beitrag Infusionstherapie 25: 142–160 (Karger, Basel)
10. Oriot D, Wood C, Gottesmann R, Huault G (1991) Severe lactic acidosis related to acute thiamine deficiency. JPEN 15: 105–109
11. Pang JA, Yardumian A, Davies R (1986) Shoshin beriberi: an underdiagnosed condition. Intensive Care Med 12: 380–383
12. Stryer L (1988) Biochemistry. Freeman, New York

Korrespondenz: Dr. Ch. Madl, Intensivstation, Universitätsklinik für Innere Medizin IV, Währinger Gürtel 18–20, A-1090 Wien, Österreich

Einfluß der Zytokine auf den Stoffwechsel

F. Stockenhuber, A. Kranz, Ch. Zauner, R. Apsner, L. Kramer,
Ch. Madl, K. Ratheiser, B. Schneeweiß und K. Lenz

Intensivstation, Universitätsklinik für Innere Medizin IV,
Allgemeines Krankenhaus, Wien, Österreich

Unter den vielen aus Plasma und Geweben stammenden Sepsis-
Mediatoren wird seit einigen Jahren den sogenannten Cytokinen
erhöhte Bedeutung beigemessen. Unter dem Namen Cytokine
wird eine Gruppe von hormonartig wirkenden Proteinen sub-
summiert, von denen früher einige unter den individuellen Namen wie Interferon, Lymphokine, Interleukin, Lymphotoxin
usw. bekannt waren. Während Hormone generell von spezia-
lisierten Organen, den endokrinen Drüsen, produziert werden
und über den Blutweg zu den jeweiligen Zielorganen gelangen,
werden Cytokine in allen Organen des Körper produziert. Sie
fungieren als „Botenstoffe" zwischen verschiedenen immunkompetenten und inflammatorisch relevanten Zellen und koor-
dinieren die Immunantwort des Körpers.

In Abb. 1 (Seite 65) wird eine Übersicht dieses Cytokinnetz-
werkes wiedergegeben.

Im folgenden soll auf die Stoffwechselveränderungen im
Rahmen der Sepsis, die direkt oder indirekt durch Zytokine mediiert sind, eingegangen werden. Grundsätzlich finden wir bei
diesem Krankheitsbild die für eine Streßreaktion typische neu-
roendokrine Antwort mit Aktivierung des zentralen und vege-
tativen Nervensystems sowie einer erhöhten Ausschüttung von
Katecholaminen, Glucagon und Cortisol. Allerdings haben
Studien an gesunden Freiwilligen gezeigt, daß durch kombinierte
Hormoninfusion die Auswirkungen auf den Stoffwechsel nicht

annähernd mit denen zu vergleichen sind, die durch eine Sepsis ausgelöst werden [1, 2]. Es hat sich deshalb zunehmend der Schwerpunkt der Studien auf die im Verlauf einer Sepsis freiwerdenden Mediatoren gerichtet. So konnte für den Tumornekrosefaktor (TNF) und für andere Zytokine wie IL-1 und IL-6 nachgewiesen werden, daß sie entweder direkt oder indirekt, d. h. über Hormone, den Stoffwechsel nachhaltig verändern [3]. Eine Zusammenfassung der Stoffwechselwirkungen nach Gabe von TNF ist in Tabelle 1 dargestellt (mod. nach Tracey et al. [3]).

Tabelle 1. Stoffwechselstörungen nach Gabe von TNF-Ergebnissen an Versuchstieren und Freiwilligen

ZNS	Fieber, Energieverbrauch ↑ Anorexie, Funktionsänderung von Hypothalamus und Hypophyse
Proteinstoffwechsel	Proteinkatabolie ↑ Proteinumsatz ↑ Ausstrom von Aminosäuren aus Muskulatur ↑ Synthese von Actin und Myosin↓
Fettstoffwechsel	Lipolyse und Fettsäurenumsatz Hypertriglyceridämie
Kohlenhydratstoffwechsel	Glucoseproduktion↑ Glucoseutilisation ↑ Glygenmobilisation ↑
Leberfunktion	Synthese von Akutphaseproteinen ↑ Aminosäuren-Aufnahme ↑ Lipogenese ↑ Lebergewicht und DNA/RNA-Gehalt ↑ Albuminsynthese ↓

Der Tumornekrosefaktor (TNF-alpha oder Cachectin) scheint in diesem Zytokinnetzwerk bei der Entwicklung der metabolischen und pathologischen Folgen der Sepsis eine sehr wesentliche Rolle zu spielen. Dies wird durch 3 Punkte untermauert.

1. Die Gabe von TNF verursacht ein Schocksyndrom und eine Gewebezerstörung, die vom Vollbild des septischen Schocks nicht zu unterscheiden ist [4].

2. Die Hemmung des TNFs in Tiermodellen mittels monoklonaler Antikörper verhindert die Entstehung des Schocks und den Tod des Tieres [5].

3. TNF kann bei Tieren und bei Menschen im septischen Schock am frühesten im Serum nachgewiesen werden. Andere Cytokine, die ebenfalls im septischen Schock eine Rolle spielen dürften wie IL-1, IL-6, IL-8 sind üblicherweise erst etwas später nachweisbar [6]. Es wird deshalb im nachfolgenden auf die Rolle des TNF im Rahmen der Cytokin mediierten Stoffwechselveränderungen besonders eingegangen.

Kohlenhydratstoffwechsel

Die wesentliche Veränderung im Kohlenhydratstoffwechsel während einer Sepsis ist die ausgeprägte Hyperglykämie, die man meist auch ohne Nährstoffzufuhr beobachten kann. Die Ursache dafür ist eine erhöhte hepatische Glucoseproduktion einerseits bedingt durch eine gesteigerte Glykogenolyse andererseits durch Gluconeogenese aus glucoplastischen Aminosäuren, Lactat, Pyruvat und Glyzerin. Die hepatische Glucoseproduktion beträgt beim Gesunden im Nüchternzustand rund 120–230 g/Tag [7], bei septischen Patienten wurden Werte um 300 g/Tag bestimmt [7]. Diese hepatische Glucoseproduktion läßt sich beim septischen Patienten auch durch Glucosegabe von ca. 400 g/Tag nicht vollständig unterdrücken.

Es ist unwahrscheinlich, daß TNF direkt die hepatische Glucoseproduktion steigern kann, da eine β-adrenerge Blockade die erhöhte Glucoseproduktion nach TNF-Infusion in Ratten vollständig verhindern konnte [8] und TNF die Gluconeogenese an isolierten Rattenhepatozyten in vitro nicht verändert [9]. Während einer Sepsis ist die Aufnahme und die Oxidation von Glucose in der Muskulatur vermindert [10]. Im Tierversuch konnte gezeigt werden, daß die Dauerinfusion von niedrig dosiertem TNF über 18 Stunden in der Ratte einen Zustand der Insulinresistenz hervorruft und die periphere Glucoseutilisation verringert [11]. Hohe Dosen von TNF verursachen jedoch Hypoglykämie, welche bei adrenalektomierten Tieren noch deutlicher ausgeprägt ist [12], sodaß TNF wahrscheinlich einen dosisabhängigen variablen Effekt auf die periphere Glucoseutilisation hat.

Fettstoffwechsel

Während einer Sepsisepisode ist der Fettumsatz deutlich erhöht. Fett wird durch erhöhte Lipolyse, hauptsächlich unter dem Einfluß der Katecholamine, aus den endogenen Depots mobilisiert und in freie Fettsäuren und Glyzerin gespalten. Dies führt zu einer verminderten Aufnahme von freien Fettsäuren und Glyzerin in der Leber. In Kombination mit der gesteigerten de novo Synthese von Fettsäuren nimmt dadurch die hepatische Produktion und die Freisetzung von Triglyzeriden zu [13, 14]. Eine Vielzahl von Studien zeigt, daß in vivo sowohl im Tierversuch als auch bei gesunden Freiwilligen eine Infusion mit TNF die Veränderungen des Fettstoffwechsels während einer Sepsis reproduzieren kann. Die Hypertriglyzeridämie nach Gabe von TNF dürfte einerseits durch Stimulation der de novo Synthese von freien Fettsäuren in der Leber [15, 16] und zweitens durch Zunahme der Reveresterung von freien Fettäuren hervorgerufen werden [15]. Eine Downregulation der Lipoproteinlipase dürfte, wenn überhaupt, nur eine untergeordnete Rolle spielen [17]. Der exakte Mechanismus durch den TNF und möglicherweise andere Cytokine wie IL-1, IL-6 und Interferon-alpha den Fettstoffwechsel verändern ist noch nicht komplett geklärt. Die hepatische Triglyzeridsynthese könnte durch TNF direkt bedingt sein, wie in vitro an Hep G 2 Zellen gezeigt werden konnte [18]. Die Rolle der Streßhormone in der Entwicklung der Hypertriglyzeridämie ist unklar. Studien in vitro zeigen, daß Glucagon und Katecholamine die VLDL Sekretion der Hepatozyten hemmen, während Glucocorticoide diese eher fördern [19]. TNF stimuliert die hepatische Lipogenese jedoch auch in adrenalektomierten Ratten, wenn auch in geringerem Umfang als in normalen Kontrolltieren [20].

Proteinstoffwechsel

Während einer Sepsisepisode sind sowohl die Synthese als auch der Abbau von Proteinen erhöht. Der Proteinabbau übertrifft jedoch die Proteinsynthese. Der daraus resultierende Nettoproteinkatabolismus äußert sich in einer negativen Stickstoffbilanz. In der Literatur werden N-Verluste von 21–37 g/Tag

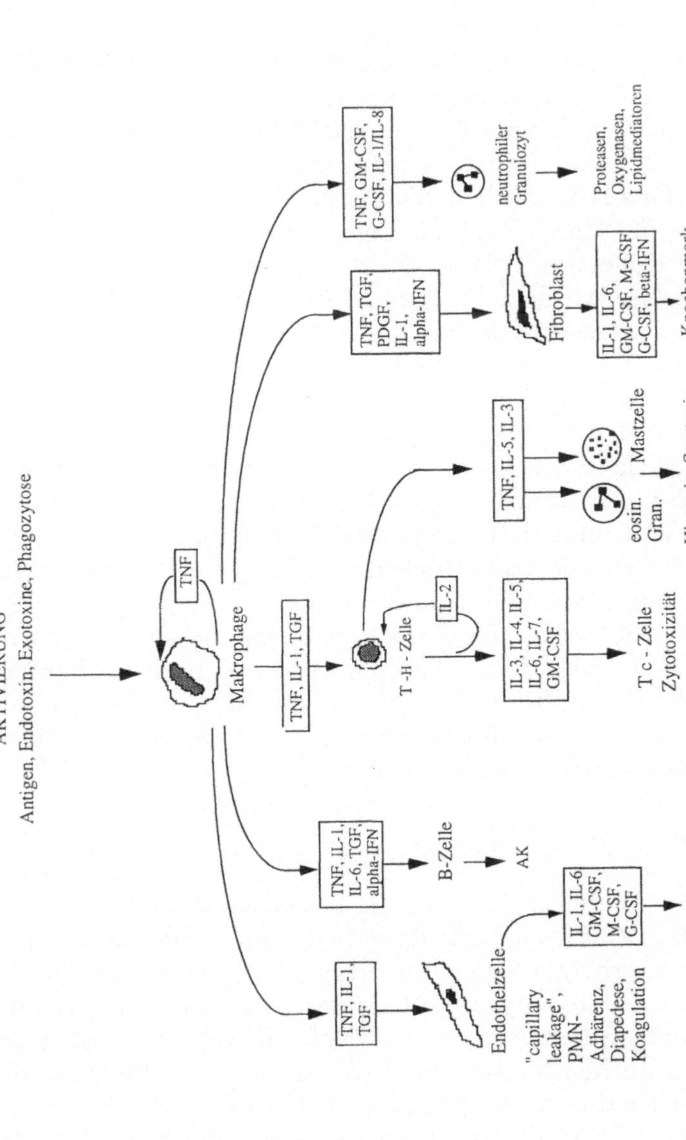

Abb. 1. Übersicht über das Zytokinnetzwerk (mod. nach Seeger [46]). Als zentraler Anteil des Zytokinnetzwerkes ist der Makrophage dargestellt. Wesentliche Wirkungen entfalten die Cytokine auf Endothelzellen, Fibroblasten, Mastzellen, zytotoxische T-Zellen (Tc-Zellen), B-Zellen und neutrophile und eosinophile Granulozyten sowie das Knochenmark

beschrieben, dies entspricht Verlusten von 500–1000 g Muskelmasse pro Tag [21]. Die zwei Hauptmerkmale im Proteinkatabolismus während der Sepsis sind die beschleunigte Proteolyse im Muskel und die erhöhte Proteinsynthese in der Leber. Dies führt zu einer beschleunigten peripheren Freisetzung von Aminosäuren, die zum Großteil in die Leber transportiert und einerseits für die Gluconeogenese und andererseits für die Synthese von Akutphaseproteinen verwendet werden. Glucocorticoide und Glucagon werden als wichtige Mediatoren für diese Veränderungen angesehen [13, 14]. Die wichtige Rolle von TNF in der durch Sepsis induzierten Muskelproteolyse wurde anhand einer Studie mit septischen Ratten erkannt, die zeigt, daß durch Gabe eines Antikörpers gegen TNF der Muskelproteinabbau weitgehend inhibiert werden kann [22]. Weitere Studien an Tiermodellen haben gezeigt, daß TNF und IL-1 eine Umverteilung von Körperproteinen bewirkt, wie sie für die Sepsis typisch ist: Stimulation der Muskelproteolyse, gleichzeitig erhöhte hepatische Proteinsynthese [23, 24, 25]. TNF und IL-1 dürften dabei auf molekulargenetischer Ebene wirken. Sie unterdrücken einerseits die Expression von m-RNA für Actin und reduzieren die Absolutmenge an 18 S und 28 S Ribosomen im Muskel, während sie andererseits die Synthese von mRNA für Akutphaseproteine in der Leber steigern [24, 26]. Teilweise jedoch dürften diese Wirkungen von TNF auf den Proteinmetabolismus durch IL-6 und Glucocorticoide mediiert werden [27, 28, 29].

Energieverbrauch

Sepsis führt zu einem Anstieg des Ruheenergieumsatzes um bis zu 60 %. Zahlreiche Faktoren wie die erhöhte Körpertemperatur, erhöhter Sauerstoffverbrauch im verletzten Gewebe, veränderte Einstellung des „Thermostaten" im Hypothalamus und erhöhter Substratumsatz von Kohlenhydraten, Lipiden und Proteinen dürften hierbei eine Rolle spielen [13]. Bei gesunden Probanden induziert TNF einen 34 % Anstieg des Ruheenergieumsatzes [30]. Weitere Faktoren, die dafür sprechen, daß TNF in diesem Zusammenhang zumindest indirekt eine Rolle spielt, sind die fieberinduzierende Wirkung von TNF und die

Aktivierung des sympathischen Nervensystems durch TNF. TNF mediiert diese Reaktion über den Cyclooxygenaseweg, da diese Wirkung im Tierversuch durch Ibuprofen blockiert werden kann [31].

Einfluß der Ernährung auf das Cytokinsystem

Die Zytokine sind primär dafür bestimmt eine Infektion zu überwinden. Erst ihre überschießende bzw. unkoordinierte Produktion löst Mechanismen aus, die schließlich zum septischen Schock führen. Die diätetische Manipulation der Zytokinbiologie kann jetzt einerseits darauf abzielen die Zytokinproduktion zu erhöhen, z. B. bei unterernährten Patienten, die eine reduzierte Syntheserate von Cytokinen aufweisen [32, 33] um die nützliche Rolle der Cytokine im Sinne einer effektiven inflammatorischen Antwort zu fördern. Sie kann aber auch darauf bedacht sein, die Cytokinaktivität zu bremsen, wenn eine verstärkte Produktion negative Auswirkungen erwarten lassen würde. Kjelden-Kragh et al. fanden, daß sich die Entzündungszeichen bei Patienten mit rheumatoider Arthritis deutlich besserten wenn sie ihre Ernährungsgewohnheiten auf vegetarische Kost umstellten. Der exakte Nährstoff, der für die Besserung der Symptome verantwortlich war, konnte nicht identifiziert werden. Die vegetarische Kost unterscheidet sich von der Omnivorenkost speziell bezüglich Fettzusammensetzung und Mikronährstoffgehalt.

Studien, die Immunantwort mit spezifischer Nahrungszufuhr zu modifizieren, konzentrierten sich besonders auf die Fettstoffe. Studien an Gesunden und an Patienten mit Entzündungszeichen haben den Einfluß von Fischöl auf die Cytokinproduktion untersucht. Die Entzündungszeichen bei rheumatoider Arthritis, Psoriasis, M. Crohn und Colitis ulcerosa konnten jeweils durch die Gabe von Fischölpräparaten gebessert werden [35, 36, 37]. Wieweit die Besserung der Symptome tatsächlich auf einer Verringerung der Cytokinproduktion zurückzuführen ist, muß jedoch offen bleiben. Endres et al. [38] konnten jedoch zeigen, daß der Konsum von 15 g Eicosapentensäure pro Tag in Form von Fischöl über 6 Wochen die IL-1 alpha und beta und TNF alpha und beta Produktion von Monozyten nach Endotoxinstimulus signifikant reduzieren. Weitere Tierstudien zeigten, daß Fischölgabe die metabolischen Veränderungen nach Endotoxinstimulus signifikant reduziert. Neben Fischöl, welches reich an w-3 mehrfach ungesättigten Fettsäuren ist, konnte auch eine Verringerung von metabolischen Effekten nach TNF Exposition durch vorangehende Verabreichung von Kokosnußöl oder Butter erzielt werden [39]. Die Wirkung von Butter war dabei deutlich stärker ausgeprägt als die von Kokosnußöl. Beide Fette sind reich an Linolsäure, Butter enthält jedoch 3,5 mal mehr einfach ungesättigte Ölsäure. Dies könnte für die unterschiedliche Wirkung verantwortlich sein [40].

Tierstudien zeigen, daß Diäten mit geringem Proteingehalt die hepatische Produktion von Akutphaseproteinen reduzieren [41]. Schwere Traumen bzw. Infektionen führen zu Veränderungen der Aminosäurenkonzentrationen im Plasma: z. B. Abfall von Glyzin, Serin und Taurin [42]. Es kommt zu einer erhöhten Utilisationsrate der schwefelhaltigen Aminosäuren Cystein und Methionin zusammen mit Glyzin und Serin um gewisse Substanzen zu produzieren wie z. B. Glutathion, die einen antioxidativen Schutz darstellen. Vor allem Cystein ist wichtig um die hepatische Produktion von Glutathion, Metallothionein sowie anderer Proteine auf TNF-Stimulation zu steigern.

Auch Vitamine dürften immunmodulatorische Wirkungen besitzen. So führt Vitamin E Mangel zu verstärkten metabolischen Reaktionen auf Endotoxinexposition. Dies dürfte auf erhöhte Cytokinproduktion durch aufgrund des Vitamin E Mangels gestörte Antioxidationsmechanismen zurückzuführen sein [43].

Vitamin A könnte ebenfalls die Cytokinproduktion beeinflussen. Es konnte gezeigt werden, daß Makrophagen von indischen Kindern, die mit 100.000 IE Vitamin A supplementiert wurden 9mal mehr IL-1 produzieren als Makrophagen einer Kontrollgruppe [44]. Schließlich dürfte auch Vitamin D eine immunmodulatorische Wirkung besitzen. Makrophagen, die mit 1,25 Dihydroxycholecalciferol behandelt wurden, produzieren größere Mengen an TNF und GM-CSF und sind effektiver Mycobacterium avium zu töten [45].

Offensichtlich ist eine Vielzahl von Nährstoffen in der Lage die Cytokinbiologie sowohl auf der Ebene der Produktion als auch auf der Ebene der Sensitivität des Erfolgsgewebes zu beeinflussen. Zukünftige Studien werden allerdings notwendig sein um das volle Ausmaß der Cytokinmodulation durch verschiedene Nährstoffe zu verstehen und um zu erkennen welche Nährstoffe tatsächlich therapeutische Potenz haben.

Literatur

1. Bessey PQ, Watters JM, Aoki TT, Wilmore DW (1984) Combined hormonal infusion stimulates the metabolic response to injury. Ann Surg 200: 264–280
2. Gelfand RA, Matthews DE, Bier DM, Sherwin RS (1984) Role of counterregulatory hormones in the catabolic response to injury. J Clin Invest 74: 2238–2248
3. Tracey KJ (1992) TNF and other cytokines in the metabolism of septic shock and cachexia. Clin Nutr 11: 1–11
4. Natanson C, Eichenholz PW, Danner RL (1989) Endotoxin and tumor necrosis factor challenges in dogs simulate the cardiovascular profile of human septic shock. J Exp Med 169: 823–832
5. Tracey KJ, Fong Y, Hesse DG (1987) Anti-cachectin/TNF monoclonal antibodies prevent septic shock during lethal bacteraemia. Nature 330: 662–664
6. Martich GD, Danner RL, Ceska M, Suffredini AF (1991) Detection of interleukin 8 and tumor necrosis factor in normal humans after intravenous endotoxin: the effect of antiinflammatory agents. J Exp Med 173: 1021–1024
7. Shangraw RE, Jahoor F, Miyoshi H, Neff WA, Stuart CA, Herndon DN, Wolfe RR (1989) Differentiation between septic and postburn insulin resistance. Metabolism 38: 983–989
8. Bagby GJ, Lang CH, Skrepnik N, Spitzer JJ (1992) Attenuation of glucose metabolic charges resulting from TNF-alpha administration by adrenergic blockade. Am J Physiol 262: R 628–635
9. Rofe AM, Conyers RAJ, Bais R, Gamble JR, Vadas MA (1987) The effects of recombinant tumor necrosis factor (cachectin) on metabolism in isolated rat adipocyte, hepatocyte and muscle preparations. Biochem J 242: 789–792
10. Shaw JH, Wolfe RR (1987) Fatty acid and glycerol kinetics in septic patients with gastrointestinal cancer. The response to glucose infusion and parenteral feeding. Ann Surg 205: 368–376
11. Lang CH, Dobrescu C, Bagley GJ (1992) Tumor necrosis factor impairs insulin action on peripheral glucose disposal and hepatic glucose output. Endocrinology 130: 43–52
12. Chajek-Shaul T, Barash V, Weidenfeld J (1990) Lethal hypoglycemia and hypothermia induced by administration of low doses of tumor necrosis factor to adrenalectomized rats. Metab Clin Exp 39: 242–250

13. Douglas RG, Shaw JHF (1989) Metabolic response to sepsis and trauma Br J Surg 76: 115–122

14. Frayn KN (1989) Hormonal control of metabolism in trauma and sepsis. Clin Endocrinol 24: 577–599

15. Feingold KR, Adi S, Staprans I (1990) Diet affects the mechanisms by which TNF stimulates hepatic triglyceride production. Am J Physiol 259: E 177–184

16. Feingold KR, Serio MK, Adi S, Moser AH, Grunfeld C (1989) Tumor necrosis factor stimulates hepatic lipid synthesis and secretion. Endocrinology 124: 2336–2342

17. Semb H, Peterson S, Tavernier J, Olivecrona T (1987) Multiple effects of tumor necrosis factor on lipoprotein lipase in vivo. J Biol Chem 262: 8390–8394

18. Grunfeld C, Dinarello CA, Feingold KR (1991) Tumor necrosis factor alpha, Interleukin-1, and Interferon-alpha stimulate triglyceride synthesis in Hep G 2 cells. Metab Clin Exp 40: 894–898

19. Gibbons GF (1990) Assembly and secretion of hepatic very-low density lipoprotein. Biochem J 268: 1–13

20. Evans RD, Williamson DH (1991) Comparison of effects of platelet-activating factor and tumor necrosis factor alpha on lipid metabolism in adrenalectomized rats in vivo. Biochem Biophys Acta 1086: 191–196

21. Streat SS, Beddoe AH, Hill G (1987) Aggressive nutritional support does not prevent protein loss despite fat gain in septic intensive care patients. J Trauma 27: 262–266

22. Zamir O, Hasselgren PO, Kunhel SL, Frederick J, Higashiguchi T, Fischer JE (1992) Evidence that tumor necrosis factor participates in the regulation of muscle proteolysis during sepsis. Arch Surg 127: 170–174

23. Moldawer LL, Andersson C, Gelin J, Lundholm KG (1988) Regulation of food intake and hepatic protein synthesis by recombinant-derived cytokines. Am J Physiol 254: G 450–456

24. Fong Y, Moldawer LL, Marano M (1989) Cachectin/TNF or IL-1 alpha induces cachexia with redistribution of body proteins. Am J Physiol 256: R 659–665

25. Flores EA, Bistrian BR, Pomposelli JJ, Dinarello CA, Blackburn GL, Istfan NW (1989) Infusion of tumor necrosis factor/cachectin promotes muscle catabolism in the rat. A synergistic effect with interleukin 1. J Clin Invest 83: 1614–1622

26. Perlmutter DH, Dinarello CA, Punsal PI, Colten HR (1986) Cachectin/ tumor necrosis factor regulates hepatic acute phase gene expression. J Clin Invest 78: 1349–1354

27. Hall-Angeraas M, Angeraas U, Zamir O, Hasselgren PO, Fischer JE (1990) Interaction between corticosterone and tumor necrosis factor stimulated protein breakdown in rat sceletal muscle, similar to sepsis. Surgery 108: 460-466

28. Fischer JE, Hasselgren PO (1991) Cytokines and glucocorticoids in the regulation of the „hepato-sceletal muscle axis" in sepsis. Am J Surg 161: 266–271

29. Andus T, Bauer J, Gerok W (1991) Effects of cytokines on the liver. Hepatology 13: 364–375

30. Van der Poll T, Romijn JA, Endert E, Borm JJJ, Büller HR, Sauerwein HP (1991) Tumor necrosis factor mimics the metabolic response to acute infection in healthy humans. Am J Physiol 261: E 457–465

31. Evans DA, Jacobs DO, Revhang A, Wilmore DW (1989) The effects of tumor necrosis factor and their selective inhibition by ibuprofen. Ann Surg 209: 312–321

32. Keenan RA, Moldawer LL, Yang RD (1982) An altered response by peripheral leucocytes to synthesise or release leucocyte endogenous mediator in critically ill protein malnourished patients. J Lab Clin Med 100: 844–857

33. Kauffman CA, Jones PG, Kluger MJ (1988) Fever and malnutrition: endogenous pyrogen/interleukin-1 in malnourished patients. Am J Clin Nutr 44: 449–452

34. Kjeldsen-Kragh J, Hangen M, Borchgrevnik CF (1991) Controlled trial of fasting and one-year vegetarian diet in rheumatoid arthritis. Lancet 339: 899–902

35. Kremer JM, Jubiz W, Michalek A (1987) Fish oil fatty acid supplementation in active rheumatoid arthritis: a double-blinded, placebo controlled, crossover trial. Ann Int Med 106: 497–502

36. Bittner SB, Tucker WFG, Cartwright I (1988) A double-blind, randomised, placebo-controlled trial of fish oil in psoriasis. Lancet i: 378–380

37. Solomon P, Kornbluth AA, Janowitz HD (1990) Treatment of ulcerative colitis with fish oil n-3-w fatty acid: an open trial. J Clin Gastroenterol 12: 157–161

38. Endres S, Glorbani R, Kelley VE (1989) The effect of dietary supplementation with n-3 polyunsaturated fatty acids on the synthesis of IL-1 and TNF-alpha by mononuclear cells. N Engl J Med 320: 266–271

39. Bashir S, Grimble RF (1992) Modulation of metabolic effects of TNF-alpha by dietary fats. J Food Sci Nutr 43: 105–111

40. Mulroney HM, Grimble RF (1992) Oleic acid as a determinant of the differences between the suppressive effects of coconut oil and butter on responses to tumor necrosis factor-alpha in rats. Proc Nutr Soc 51

41. Jennings G, Bougeois C, Elia M (1993) The magnitude of the acute phase response is attenuated by protein deficiency in rats. J Nutr 122: 1325–1331

42. Paaw JD, Davis AT (1990) Taurine concentrations in serum of critically injured patients and age- and sex-matched healthy control subjects. Am J Clin Nutr 49: 814–822

43. Troughton K, Grimble RF (1992) Vitamin E status modulates the inflammatory response to endotoxin in rats. Proc Nutr Soc 51

44. Bhaskaram P, Sharada K, Sivakumar B (1989) Effect of iron and vitamin A deficiences on macrophage function in children. Nutr Rev 9: 35–45

45. Bermudez LEM, Young LS, Gupta S (1990) 1, 25 Dihydroxy vitamin D 3-dependent inhibition of growth or killing of Mycobacterium avium complex in human macrophages is mediated by TNF and GM-CSF. Cell Immunol 127: 432–441
46. Seeger W, Grimminger F, Walmrath D (1993) Mediatorblockade (Mediatorinhibitoren, -antagonisten, -antikörper). In: Schuster HP (Hrsg) Intensivtherapie bei Sepsis und Multiorganversagen. Springer, Berlin Heidelberg New York Tokyo

Korrespondenz: Doz. Dr. F. Stockenhuber, Intensivstation, Klinik für Innere Medizin IV, Universität Wien, Währinger Gürtel 18–20, A-1090 Wien, Österreich

Therapie der Azidose bei Sepsis

K. Lenz

Intensivstation, Klinik für Innere Medizin IV,
Universität Wien, Österreich

Die Ursache der Azidose im Rahmen einer schweren Sepsis,
bzw. septischen Schocks besteht einerseits in einer intrazellulären Akkumulation von H+ Ionen vorwiegend aus der
ATP Hydrolyse (metabolische Azidose), einer verminderten
renalen Elimination bei Nierenversagen (metabolische Azidose) und bei zusätzlich schwerster respiratorischer Insuffizienz
in einer verminderten CO_2 Elimination (respiratorische Azidose).

Ziel jeder Therapie muß es sein primär die Ursache zu beseitigen. Dies würde bedeuten: Eine Verbesserung des Stoffwechsels mit einer Erhöhung der Umwandlung von Pyruvat in
AcetylCoA und damit Verbesserung der Glukoseoxidation mit
einer effizienteren Energiegewinnung, einer vermehrten Elimination durch Verwendung extrakorporaler Systeme (Hämo-
dialyse, Hämofiltration) und Verbesserung der Beatmung ev.
mit zusätzlicher extrakorporaler CO_2 Elimination (Tabelle 1).

Tabelle 1. Therapie der Ursache

Thiamin 600 mg i.v.
Dichloroazetat 50 mg/kg i.v.
Extrakorporale Therapien

Eine Normalisierung der Glukoseoxydation kann bis zu einem
gewissen Grade durch Gabe von Thiamin einem CoEnzym der
Pyruvatdehydrogenase erzielt werden. V. a. bei chronisch unterernährten Patienten kann der Thiaminmangel relevante Aus-

maße annehmen und durch die Gabe von Thiamin eine pH Anhebung und Laktatabnahme erzielt werden [9].

Dichloroazetat führt ebenfalls zu einer Verbesserung der Glukoseoxidation über Stimulation der Pyruvatdehydrogenase, sowie zu einer Hemmung der Glukoseoxydation. Daraus resultiert eine Verminderung der Laktatproduktion. Diese Verminderung der Laktatkonzentration ging im Endotoxinschock jedoch nicht mit einer Verbesserung der Überlebensrate einher [15].

Auch in einer klinischen Studie konnte zwar eine Besserung des pH Wertes und des Laktates, nicht jedoch ein Einfluß auf die Prognose gesehen werden [14].

Während die Beherrschung der Ursache einer metabolischen Azidose im Rahmen einer Sepsis allgemein anerkannt ist, ist die symptomatische Therapie der Azidose mit Puffersubstanzen umstritten. Nicht klar ist inwiefern eine Azidose eventuell sogar günstig auf den Verlauf ist, bzw. bei welchem pH-Wert eine Therapie einsetzen soll. Die tierexperimentellen Untersuchungen hierzu sind widersprüchlich [2, 3, 5, 12]. Derzeit stehen 3 Puffersubstanzen zur klinischen Anwendung zur Verfügung: Natriumbikarbonat, THAM und Carbicarb (Tabelle 2). Mit allen 3 Substanzen kann der pH-Wert angehoben werden, klinische Studien über einen positiven Effekt dieser Substanzen hinsichtlich Morbidität und Mortalität fehlen jedoch bislang.

Tabelle 2. Symptomatische Therapie

| THAM |
| Na Bikarbonat |
| Carbicarb |

Tabelle 3. Physikochemische Eigenschaften

	NaBikarbonat	Carbicarb	THAM	
Na^+	1000	1000	0	mmol/L
HCO_3^-	1000	333	0	mmol/L
CO_3^{2-}	0	333	0	mmol/L
pH (25° C)	8,3	9,6	10,3	
Osmolalität	2000	1667	350	mOsm/kg

THAM (Trishydroxymethylaminomethan)

ist ein Aminoalkohol. Die Osmolarität und der Natriumload ist geringer als vergleichsweise durch Gabe von NaBikarbonat.

$$H_2O + CO_2 > H_2CO_3 > THAM\ H^+ + HCO_3^-$$
$$THAM$$

Die Reaktion ist nach rechts verschoben, sodaß CO_2 eliminiert und Bikarbonat produziert wird. Dieser CO_2 mindernde Effekt steht im Gegensatz zu den Auswirkungen einer Na-Bikarbonattherapie, bei der CO_2 gebildet wird. Durch THAM ist daher auch eine intrazelluläre pH-Anhebung zu erwarten, diese führte tierexperimentell zu einem positiv inotropen Effekt am ischämischen Myokard [4]. Der Nachteil von THAM ist die vergleichsweise sehr hohe Toxizität mit Schädigung von Hepatozyten und Tubuluszellen, v. a. wenn die Elimination im Rahmen des Schockes nicht gegeben ist. Weiters darf die Substanz nur über einen zentralvenösen Katheter infundiert werden. Als Tagesmaximaldosis werden 4,2 mmol/kg KG empfohlen, die Infusionsgeschwindigkeit mit 0,1 mmol/kg/min.

Natriumbikarbonat

Die NaBikarbonatgabe führt zu einer Erhöhung von CO_2 (H^+ und HCO_3^- gehen in H_2O und CO_2 über). CO_2 kann leicht in die Zelle diffundieren und dort durch Verbindung mit H_2O zu einer Verstärkung der intrazellulären Azidose führen. In experimentellen Arbeiten konnte eine Abhängigkeit der Verschlechterung der Linksventrikelfunktion vom pCO_2 bei Azidose gezeigt werden. Dies wurde auf die Verschlechterung der intrazellulären Azidose zurückgeführt [12]. Klinisch dürften jedoch hohe pCO_2 Werte keine Rolle spielen, wie die Untersuchungen mit der permissive Hyperkapnie zeigen, bei denen pCO_2 Werte über 100 mmHg problemlos toleriert werden [6].

In klinischen Vergleichsstudien – NaBikarbonat gegen 0,9 % NaCl – konnte durch die Gabe von NaBikarbonat eine Anhebung des pH gesehen werden, nicht jedoch Auswirkungen auf die Hämodynamik, DO2 oder VO2 und Laktat [10, 11]. Der myokardiale Sauerstoffverbrauch nahm bei Patienten mit con-

gestiver CMP durch Abnahme der Extraktion und des Ange-
botes ab [1].

Carbicarb

Besteht aus Natriumcarbonat (Na_2CO_3) und Natriumbicarbonat
($NaHCO_3$) zu äquimolaren Teilen.

$$CO_3^- + CO_2 + H_2O > 2\ HCO_3^-$$
$$\updownarrow$$
$$H^+ + HCO_3^-$$

Da der CO_2 bindende Effekt das aus dem Bikarbonat gebildete CO_2 neutralisiert ergibt sich bei Carbicarb im Unterschied zu NaBikarbonat keine oder nur eine minimale CO_2
Nettogeneration. Daraus wurde ein möglicher Vorteil gegenüber
NaBikarbonat abgeleitet.

In tierexperimentellen Untersuchungen war der Effekt Carbicarb gegenüber NaBikarbonat entweder gleich bezogen auf
den intramyokardialen pH und Hämodynamik [13] oder besser
bezogen auf Blutdruck und EEG [7].

In einer prospektiven Studie an 36 postoperativen Patienten
mit metabolischer Azidose wurde nach Carbicarb ein höheres
HZV (p = 0,048), eine verbesserte Laktatutilization (p = 0,033)
ein niedrigerer PCWP (p = 0,012) und ein erniedrigtes 2,3 DPG
(p = 0,045) gefunden [8].

Zusammenfassung

Die Therapie der metabolischen Azidose bei Patienten mit Sepsis
umfaßt in erster Linie die Ursache zu beherrschen. Der Einsatz
von alkalisierenden Substanzen ist bislang umstritten. Mit den
erhältlichen Substanzen kann der pH Wert angehoben werden,
ein Einfluß auf die Morbidität und Mortalität konnte bislang
nicht nachgewiesen werden. Es konnte aber auch nicht nachgewiesen werden, daß einer der Substanzen negative Effekt
ausüben würde, da der experimentell nachgewiesene ungünstige
Effekt einer erhöhten CO_2 Produktion klinisch bislang nicht
bestätigt wurde.

Literatur

1. Bersin RM, Chatterjee K, Arieff Al (1989) Metabolic and hemodynamic consequences of sodium bicarbonate administration in patients with heart disease. Am J Med 87: 7–14
2. Cingolani HE, Faulkner SL, Mattiazzis AR, Bender HW, Graham TP (1975) Depression of human myocardial contractility with respiratory and metabolic acidosis. Surgery 77: 427–432
3. Davies AO (1984) Rapid desensitization and uncoupling of human β-adrenergic receptors in an in vitro model of lactic acidosis. J Clin Endocrinol Metabol 59: 398–405
4. Effron MB, Guarnieri T, Frederiksen JW, Greene HL, Weisfeldt ML (1978) Am J Physiol 235: H 167–174
5. Gores GG, Nieminen AL, Wray BE, Herman B, Lemasters JJ (1989) Intracellular pH during „Chemical Hypoxia" in cultured rat hepatocytes. Protection by intracellular acidosis against onset of cell death. J Clin Invest 83: 386–396
6. Hickling KG, Henderson SJ, Jackson R (1980) Low mortality associated with low volume pressure limited ventilation with permissive hypercapnia in severe adult respiratory distress syndrome. Intensive Care Med 16: 372–377
7. Kucera R, Whalen W, Shapiro JI (1991) Electroenzephalographic consequences of alkalanization therapy during lactic acisosis: different effects of sodium bicarbonate and carbicarb. J Crit Care 6: 71–74
8. Landow L, Leung J, Heard SO, Franke M, Mangano D, Arieff Al (1993) Prospective randomized double blind multicenter study of $NaHCO_3$ versus Carbicarb in the treatment of metabolic acidosis. Anesth Analg k76: S 205
9. Madl C, Kranz A, Liebisch B, Traindl O, Lenz K, Druml W (1993) Lactic acidosis in thiamine deficiency. Clin Nutr 12: 108–111
10. Mark NH, Leund JM, Arieff Al, Mangano DT (1993) Safety of low-dose intraoperative bicarbonate therapy: a prospective, double-blind, randomized study. Crit Care Med 21: 659–665
11. Mathieu D, Neviere R, Billard V, Fleyfel M, Wattel F (1991) Effects of bicarbonate therapy on hemodynamics and tissue oxygenation in patients with lactic acidosis: a prospective, controlled clinical study. Crit Care Med 19: 1352–1356
12. Ng M, Levy ML, Zieske HA (1967) Effects of changes of pH and of carbon dioxide tension on left ventricular performance. Am J Physiol 213: 115–120
13. Sonett J, Baker LS, Hsi C, Knox MA, Visner MS, Landow L (1993) Sodium bicarbonate versus carbicarb in canine myocardial hypercarbic acidosis. J Crit Care 8: 1–11
14. Stapcoole PW, Wright EC, Baumgartner TG, Bersin RM, Buchhalter S, Curry SH, Duncan CA, Harman EM, Lorenz A, Schneider SH, Siegel JH, Summer WR, Thompson D, Wolfe CL, Zorovich B (1992) A controlled

trial of dichloroacetate for treatment of lactic acidosis in adults. N Engl J Med 327: 1564–1569

15. Weingad KW, Fettman MJ, Philips RW, Hand MS (1986) Metabolic effects of sodium dichloroacetae in endotoxemic minipigs. Circ Chock 19: 55–67

Korrespondenz: Prof. Dr. K. Lenz, Intensivstation, Klinik für Innere Medizin IV, Währinger Gürtel 18–20, A-1090 Wien, Österreich

Therapie der Stoffwechselstörungen bei Sepsis:
Pharmakologische Beeinflussung

E. Roth

Chirurgisches Stoffwechselforschungslabor,
Klinik für Chirurgie, Universität Wien, Österreich

„Metabolic care of the critically ill" ist der Titel eines von D. Wilmore geschriebenen Buches, das 1975 erschien [1]. In diesem Buch beschreibt Wilmore die Stoffwechselveränderungen und die daraus abzuleitenden therapeutischen Maßnahmen beim Intensivpatienten. Als primäre therapeutische Stoffwechseltherapie wird in diesem Buch vor allem eine gezielte parenterale Ernährung angesehen. Das Spektrum der Stoffwechseltherapie hat sich in den letzten Jahren wesentlich erweitert, und wir befinden uns zur Zeit diesbezüglich in einer faszinierenden Phase von neuen Erkenntnissen, wobei vor allem die Entdeckung der Zytokine/Wachstumsfaktoren und das Verstehen der Kreislaufregulation über das einfache Molekül Stickoxid (NO) zu vermerken sind.

Die Stoffwechselsituation beim septischen Patienten wird als Postaggressionssyndrom (-stoffwechsel) bezeichnet. Dieser unterscheidet sich ganz wesentlich vom Stoffwechsel im gesunden Zustand. Charakterisiert ist der Postaggressionszustand durch ein kataboles Zustandsbild mit einem vermehrten Abbau von Skelettmuskulatur und Fett und einem erhöhten Plasmaglukosespiegel aufgrund einer verschlechterten peripheren Insulinwirkung.

Teleologische Betrachtung über eine pharmakologische Stoffwechseltherapie bei Sepsis

Bevor wir an eine Stoffwechseltherapie bei septischen Patienten denken, müssen wir uns fragen, inwieweit das pathogene Stoffwechselgeschehen als gewünschte Reaktion auf die Krankheit zu sehen ist und ob diese Stoffwechselveränderungen primär nicht dazu dienen, bei kritisch Erkrankten lebenswichtige Organfunktionen auf Kosten nicht so wichtiger aufrecht zu erhalten. Das beste Beispiel hierfür ist der Eiweißkatabolismus, also der Verlust an Skelettmuskulatur (Übersicht: [2]). Teleologisch gesehen, dient dieser Verlust dazu, den beim kritisch Erkrankten nicht unbedingt notwendigen Skelettmuskel abzubauen, also Stickstoff in Form von Aminosäuren vom Muskel zu exportieren und diese in das Splanchnikumgebiet weiterzuleiten. Hier werden, nach dem jetzigen Stand des Wissens, diese Aminosäuren für zwei Hauptfunktionen verwendet: Einerseits zur Energiegewinnung und andererseits zur Neusynthese von Proteinen, die den Krankheitsverlauf hemmen können. So wird Glutamin nach Transaminierung direkt vom Darm zur Energieverwertung verwendet. Aus den glukoneogenetischen Aminosäuren entsteht Glukose, die zur Energieversorgung des Zentralnervensystems dient. Ein anderer Teil der Aminosäuren wird für die hepatische Proteinsynthese zum Aufbau von Akutphasenproteinen verwendet. Glukose, Aminosäuren und Proteine sind aber auch notwendig für die Wundheilung, so daß zu ersehen ist, daß der Skelettmuskel auch als Reserveorgan für Regenerationsprozesse dient. Newsholm hat hier der Sinnhaftigkeit des Eiweißkatabolismus einen weiteren Mosaikstein hinzugefügt. Er bezeichnet in einer seiner Arbeiten den Skelettmuskel als Reserveorgan der Immunologie, da das vom Muskel freigesetzte Glutamin als essentielles Substrat für die Proliferation von rasch wachsenden Immunzellen wie Lymphozyten, Monozyten und Granulozyten gebraucht wird [3].

Obwohl schon 1981 von unserer Arbeitsgruppe ein extrem erniedrigter Glutaminspiegel bei septischen Patienten beschrieben wurde [4], haben erst jüngst erschienene Arbeiten von Häussinger eine Erklärung angeboten, warum die Zelle den Glutaminspiegel erniedrigt. Häussinger und Mitarbeiter haben an Leberzellen gezeigt, daß Aminosäuren wesentlich an der Regulation des Zellvolumens beteiligt sind [5]. Ein kleines Zellvolumen stimuliert katabole Vorgänge, wohingegen eine Vergrößerung des Zellvolumens eine Vermehrung der anabolen Vorgänge bedeutet. In einer jüngst erschienenen Publikation stellten wir die Hypothese auf, daß beim kritisch erkrankten Patienten der Eiweißkatabolismus (ausgedrückt über die Stickstoffbilanz) in Korrelation zu einer Verkleinerung des Zellvolumens steht [6]. Eiweißkatabolie und Zellvolumen korrelieren invers mit der intrazellulären Glutaminkonzentration des Skelettmuskels. Man könnte daraus schließen, daß die niedrige Glutaminkonzentration aus rein osmotischen Gründen zu einer Zellverkleinerung und deswegen ursächlich zu einer Stimulation abbauender Prozesse führt. Dieser Abbau des Skelettmuskels unterstützt eine Reihe von metabolischen Funktionen in lebenswichtigen Organen. Aus dem hier angeführten Beispiel des Eiweißkatabolismus läßt sich ableiten, daß der Erfolg einer pharmakologischen Therapie beim septischen Patienten nicht als Therapie eines Einzelphänomens gesehen werden kann. Eine objektive Beurteilung ist letztlich nur über eine Verbesserung der Prognose der septischen Patienten möglich. Dieser Nachweis gelingt bei einem derart komplizierten Krankengut, wie es der septische Patient darstellt, nur über große Multizenterstudien. Wir werden sehen, daß sich der an kleinen Kollektiven gezeigte Erfolg einiger pharmakologischer Stoffwechseltherapien, in Multizenterstudien, die auf eine Verbesserung der Mortalität ausgerichtet waren, nicht reproduzieren ließ.

Glutamin, Glutaminpeptide

Wie im vorangestellten Kapitel festgehalten, kommt es bei septischen Patienten zu einem beträchtlichen intrazellulären Glutaminmangel im Skelettmuskel, der mit der Prognose der Patienten korreliert [4]. Die Aminosäure Glutamin hat eine Reihe von wichtigen physiologischen Aufgaben inne. Publikationen zeigten Glutamin als wichtiges energetisches Substrat des Darms, als Stimulator der Immunantwort, als Regulator des Säure-Basehaushalts, als Stimulator der Proteinsynthese (in einer hormonähnlichen Wirkung), als Wirkstoff gegen die Translokation der Bakterien vom Darm zur Leber und als essentielles Substrat für alle rasch proliferierenden Zellpopulationen des Körpers. Man könnte verallgemeinernd Glutamin als anabol wirkendes Substrat bezeichnen [7].

Obwohl Glutamin die quantitativ bedeutendste freie Aminosäure des Körpers ist, kommt sie in parenteralen Nährlösungen nicht vor, da sie in wäßrigen Lösungen instabil ist und sie in Ammoniak und toxisches Pyroglutamat zerfällt. Die Gabe von stabilem Glutamat (Glutaminsäure) oder alpha-Ketoglutarat führt zu keiner Steigerung des Glutaminspiegels im Plasma [8]. In den USA versucht man Glutamin in parenteralen Nährlösungen anzubieten, indem eine tägliche Zubereitung der Lösung erfolgen soll bzw. Glutaminlösungen über eine geschlossene Kühlkette angeliefert werden soll [7]. Wesentlich gangbarer (aber teurer) ist die Verwendung von glutaminhältigen Dipeptiden (Alanylglutamin oder Glyzylglutamin), die in wäßrigen Lösungen stabil sind. Glutamin wird sehr rasch verstoffwechselt, und die Wirksamkeit von Glutamin (oder Glutamindipeptiden) auf den Stoffwechsel bzw. auf immunologische Vorgänge konnte bis jetzt nur dann nachgewiesen werden, wenn Glutamin in pharmakologischen Dosen verabreicht wurde. Die Gabe von Glutamin bei Sepsis verringert die Glutaminfreisetzung vom Muskel, scheint allerdings bei septischen Patienten das intrazelluläre Glutamindefizit nicht nachhaltig zu verringern [11].

Antikörper und Antagonisten gegen Bakterientoxine und Sepsismediatoren

Mit der Erkenntnis, daß allein die intravenöse Gabe von Endotoxin die Bildung einer Kaskade von Mediatoren mit Peptidcharakter hervorruft und diese Mediatoren eine Beeinträchtigung von Organfunktionen bewirken, begann man den Zusammenhang von Zytokinwirkung und Sepsis zu studieren. Diese Mediatoren wurden Zytokine oder Interleukine genannt, da ihre Synthese spezifisch in bestimmten Zellpopulationen abläuft und sie in autokriner Weise das Wachstum anderer Zellen beeinflussen. Die für das septische Krankheitsgeschehen bedeutendsten sind vor allem der Tumornekrosefaktor (TNF), auch Kachektin genannt, und das Interleukin-1 (IL-1). Als vielversprechende Sepsistherapie erscheint zur Zeit neben einer Anti-Endotoxintherapie eine Blockierung dieser beiden Zytokine. Über dieses Thema gibt es eine Reihe von neuen Reviews, wobei in unserem Sprachraum vor allem der jüngst von K. Werdan veröffentlichte zu erwähnen ist [12, 13]. Wenn man die bis jetzt vorliegenden Ergebnisse über Therapien mit Antizytokinen- bzw. Antiendotoxinen darstellt, muß darauf hingewiesen werden, daß zur Zeit eine Reihe von prospektiven klinischen Versuchen laufen, die die bis jetzt vorliegenden Ergebnisse in Frage stellen können.

Bis jetzt liegen die Ergebnisse von zwei Studien mit unterschiedlichen Antikörpern gegen Endotoxin vor. Eine Studie wurde mit einem humanen Antikörper (HA-1A), und eine andere mit einem murinen monoklonalen IgM Antikörpers (E5) durchgeführt [14, 15]. Mit keinem der beiden Antikörper konnte mit dem Einschlußkriterium „Sepsis mit Verdacht auf gramnegative Infektion" die Sterblichkeit im Gesamtkollektiv signifikant gesenkt werden. HA-1A verbesserte allerdings die Überlebensrate in einer der drei gebildeten Untergruppierungen, nämlich in Patienten mit einer gramnegativen Bakteriämie.

Die Wirkung von Zytokinen kann mittels spezifischer Antikörper oder über endogen gebildete Faktoren blockiert werden. Zytokine induzieren beim Menschen eine klassische Streßhormonantwort. Endogen gebildete, hemmende Substanzen gegen TNF-a oder IL-6 haben einen proteinogenen Charakter. Die Wirkung von TNF-a wird mittels spezifischer Rezeptormoleküle blockiert, wohingegen die inhibitorischen Proteine gegenüber Interleukin-1 als kompetitiv gegenüber den Rezeptorproteinen für Interleukin-1 zu verstehen sind. Es ist bereits geglückt, eine Sequenzanalyse dieser Rezeptorenproteine von TNF durchzuführen, und wir sprechen heute von einem TNF-Typ-I und einem TNF-Typ-II-Rezeptor [16]. Es ist darauf hinzuweisen, daß die Halbwertszeit dieser löslichen TNF-Rezeptoren extrem kurz ist und im Bereich von Minuten liegt.

Tierexperimentelle Studien mit einem monoklonalen Antikörper gegen TNF-a/Kachektin haben gezeigt, daß Tiere die mit diesem Antikörper immunisiert wurden, eine geringere Hypotension entwickeln als die Kontrollgruppen [17]. Allerdings muß dazu gesagt werden, daß der neutralisierende Antikörper vor der bakteriellen Infizierung gegeben wurde. Zur Zeit sind große multizentrische Studien in den USA und in Europa im Gange, die die Wirksamkeit von TNF-Antikörper als Sepsistherapeutikum zeigen sollen.

Neutralisierende Antikörper gegen Interleukin-1-β verringern das durch Endotoxin induzierte Fieber bei Tieren und verringern die Proliferation von Leukozyten [18]. Als therapeutisches Prinzip gegen die Wirkung von Interleukin-1 versucht man Antagonisten gegen den Interleukin-1 Rezeptor zu verwenden. Dieses biologisch vorkommende Molekül kommt im Plasma von gesunden Personen nicht vor, wird allerdings in den Hautkeratinozyten und in neuralen Zellen gefunden. Tierversuche haben gezeigt, daß die Gabe von Interleukin-1-Rezeptorantagonisten die Schwere der Entzündungsprozesse verringert [19]. In einer Phase-II-Studie bei Patienten mit Sepsissyndrom und Hypotension und/oder Organdysfunktion konnte durch die Gabe des Interleukin-1-Rezeptorantagonisten die Sterblichkeit dosisabhängig von 44 % in der Placebogruppe auf minimal 16 % in der Verumgruppe gesenkt werden [20]. Dieser Effekt, der bei einer Studie mit 99 Patienten gezeigt wurde, konnte in einer nachfolgenden Phase-III-Studie an 893 Patienten nicht reproduziert werden, da die Sterblichkeit in der Therapiegruppe und der Kontrollgruppe nicht signifikant unterschiedlich war [21].

Wachstumshormon/Wachstumsfaktoren als anabole Stimulatoren

Das Wachstumshormon ist das bedeutendste Hormon des Hypophysenvorderlappens. Es wurde schon 1961 auf seine anabole Wirksamkeit bei schwerverbrannten Patienten untersucht [22]. Durch den Fortschritt der Gentechnik ist es heute möglich, rekombinantes Wachstumshormon in großen Mengen herzustellen. Bei verschiedenen Spezies und unterschiedlichsten Bedingungen konnte gezeigt werden, daß das Wachstumshormon eine Stickstoffretention bewirkt. Neben dieser anabolen Wirkung auf den Stickstoffhaushalt beeinflußt das Wachstumshormon auch den Fett- und Kohlenhydratstoffwechsel. Ein Teil der anabolen Effekte des Wachstumshormons erfolgt über Somatomedine. Die wichtigsten Vertreter der Somatomedine sind der Insulin-Like Growth Factor-I (IGF-I) und Insulin-Like Growth Factor-II (IGF-II). Verschiedene Studien haben gezeigt, daß das Wachstumshormon bei katabolen Patienten einen stickstoffretinierenden Effekt hat. So verbesserte die Gabe von Wachstumshormon die Stickstoffbilanz bei internistischen Patienten und nach selektiven chirurgischen Eingriffen [23, 24]. Unterschiedliche Ergebnisse wurden beim kritisch erkrankten Patienten publiziert. Die Wirkung des Wachstums- hormon bei diesen Patienten scheint von der Stoffwechselsituation des Patienten abzuhängen. Die bis jetzt vorliegenden Studien vermitteln den Eindruck, als ob Wachstumshormon in der akuten katabolen Phase keinen anabolen Effekt hat [25, 26], jedoch in der Rekonvaleszenzphase die anabolen Vorgänge beschleunigt. Eigene Untersuchungen bei polytraumatisierten Patienten zeigten, daß die Gabe von Wachstumshormon während der ersten 7 Tage nach dem Trauma, keine Verbesserung der Stickstoffbilanz brachte [27]. Unbeeinflußt blieben auch die Konzentrationen der bestimmten Plasmaproteine (Albumin, Präalbumin, retinolbindendes Protein) obwohl Wachstumshormon die Sekretion von IGF-I gefördert hat [27]. Es hat den Anschein, als ob hier die Wirksamkeit des Wachstumshormons durch die katabolen Hormone beeinträchtigt ist. Eine jüngst erschienene Studie bei septischen Patienten beschreibt eine Verbesserung der Stickstoffbilanz von –3,7 g in der Kontrollgruppe auf 1,2 g in der mit Wachstumshormon behandelten Gruppe [28]. Bei dieser Studie ist allerdings zu vermerken, daß die Stickstoffbilanz der septischen Patienten mit ungefähr –4 ± 4 g wesentlich positiver ist, als sie sich in anderen Studien darstellt.

Untersuchungen bei Intensivpatienten haben gezeigt, daß die Konzentration des Insulin-Like Growth Factors trotz eines normalen oder selbst erhöhten Wachstumshormonspiegels signifikant erniedrigt ist [29]. Die Gabe von Insulin Like Growth Factor-I an Mäuse und Ratten im hyperkatabolen Zustand, brachte eine Verbesserung der Gewichtszunahme. Positive Ergebnisse wurden auch bei Patienten nach großen gastrointestinalen Eingriffen gezeigt. Hier brachte die einmalige Gabe von IGF-I eine Senkung des Serumcholesterinspiegels und ein Absinken des Kreatinins [30]. Es gibt allerdings auch Studien, bei denen IGF-I keinen anabolen Effekt gezeigt hat [31]. In einer eigenen Untersuchung in einem katabolen Hundemodell konnten wir zeigen, daß die Gabe von IGF-I die Stickstofffreisetzung vom Skelettmuskel nicht reduzierte, wohl aber die Aminosäureaufnahme der Leber stimulierte [32]. Es ist zu vermerken, daß sowohl für die Gabe von Wachstumshormon als auch für die Gabe von Insulin Like Growth Factor entsprechende multizentrische Studien noch ausständig sind, die eine Wirksamkeit dieser beiden anabolen Substanzen beim kritisch erkrankten Patienten nachweisen.

Arginin, Stickoxid (NO) und Argininanaloga

Obwohl die vasodilatierenden Effekte von Nitraten seit langem bekannt sind, ist der Wirkungsmechanismus dieser Substanzen erst jüngst aufgeklärt worden (Übersicht: [33, 34]). Als verantwortliches Molekül für die vasodilatierende Wirkung wurde Stickoxid (NO) erkannt, das im Endothel gebildet wird und dem Endothel-Relaxing-Factor (EDRF) gleichzusetzen ist. In der Zwischenzeit haben wir gelernt, daß NO von einer Reihe von unterschiedlichen Zellen gebildet wird und vor allem aus Arginin synthetisiert wird. Das für die NO-Synthese verantwortliche Enzym aus Arginin ist die NO-Synthase, wobei es hier ein konstitutives Enzym gibt, und eines, das über Endotoxin und Interleukine stimulierbar ist. Die NO-Bildung aus dem letzteren scheint für die septische Stoffwechselsituation von besonderer Bedeutung zu sein, da die vermehrte, induzierte NO-Bildung die Ursache der Hypotension sein könnte und außerdem eine vermehrte NO-Bildung sowohl die hepatische Proteinsynthese als auch den oxidativen Zellstoffwechsel hemmen kann. Therapieversuche laufen zur Zeit über die Verabreichung von Argininantagonisten, wie N-Monomethyl-L-Arginin (L-NMMA), N-Nitro-L-Arginin-Methylester (l-NAME) oder N-Nitro-L-Arginin. Erste Ergebnisse bei septischen Patienten, die mit N-Nitro-L-Arginin behandelt wurden, lassen schließen, daß die Hemmung der NO-Bildung mittels Argininanaloga bedeutende hämodynamische und pulmonale Veränderungen bewirken kann [35]. So kommt es unter der Gabe von N-Nitro-

L-Arginin zu einem signifikanten Anstieg des Blutdruckes (von 89 auf 140 mm Hg) und zu einer gleichzeitigen Senkung des Cardiac Index. Alle diese Veränderungen durch NNA werden durch die Gabe von L-Arginin rückgängig gemacht. Der Argininstoffwechsel dürfte auch teilweise für das Reperfusionssyndrom nach Lebertransplantation verantwortlich sein, da eigene Untersuchungen gezeigt haben, daß es unmittelbar nach Revaskularisierung zu einem systemischen Argininmangel aufgrund einer vermehrten Arginasefreisetzung kommt [36].

Der Ergänzung halber sei noch erwähnt, daß es neben den bis jetzt besprochenen pharmakologischen Thrapeutika, noch Therapieansätze mit Komponenten, die das Komplement- oder Gerinnungssystem betreffen, wie das Bradykinin, den C1-Inhibitor oder den plättchenaktivierenden Faktor (PAF). Auch Komponenten des Prostaglandinsystems bzw. Sauerstoffradikalfänger zählen zu möglichen Pharmaka gegen die Stoffwechselveränderung bei Sepsis. Aus Platzgründen kann auf diese Substanzen aber nicht eingegangen werden.

Zusammenfassend möchte ich feststellen, daß nach der Entdeckung der Zytokine als neue hormonähnliche Regulationsschiene nun wieder vermehrt basale Stoffwechselforschung bei Sepsis betrieben wird. Es ist zu erwarten, daß zukünftige Untersuchungen sich wiederum den Stoffwechselveränderungen am zellulären Niveau orientieren. Es ist nach wie vor faszinierend und nicht aufgeklärt, warum die chirurgische Sanierung eines septischen Herdes zu einer schlagartigen Verbesserung der metabolischen Situation beim Patienten führt. Nach isolierter Betrachtung der Nichtfunktion einzelner Organsysteme (ARDS) erkennt man heute immer mehr, daß Sepsis gleichzusetzen ist mit einem „Andersfunktionieren" aller Zellsysteme im Sinne eines Zellversagens. Eine Schlüsselrolle spielt hier möglicherweise eine verminderte Verstoffwechselung des Sauerstoffs, da es in der Sepsis trotz eines ausreichenden Sauerstoffangebotes im Gewebe zu einer Verminderung der oxidativen Prozesse kommt [37]. Abschließend sei noch ein interessanter Zusammenhang aufgezeigt, der die Stoffwechselwege von den Zytokinen bis zur Proteinsynthese und dem oxidativen Metabolismus verbindet. Es wurde nämlich gezeigt, daß in der Sepsis die NO-Synthese prinzipiell erhöht ist [38]. Die NO-Synthese wird durch Zytokine stimuliert [39]. Eine vermehrte NO-Bildung hemmt aber sowohl die hepatische Proteinsynthese als auch Enzyme der Atmungskette [39, 40]. Inwieweit die Gabe von gasförmigem NO zur Bekämpfung des ARDS diese negativen Effekte noch zusätzlich stimuliert, müssen zukünftige Studien zeigen.

Literatur

1. Wilmore DW (1977) The metabolic management of the criticall ill. Plenum, New York
2. Wilmore DW (1991) Catabolic illness. Strategies for enhancing recovery. N Engl J Med 325: 695–702
3. Newsholm EA, Newsholme P, Curi R, Challoner E, Ardawi MSM (1988) The role for muscle in the immune system; its importance in surgery, trauma, sepsis and burns. Nutrition 4: 261–268
4. Roth E, Funovics J, Mühlbacher F, Schemper M, Mauritz W, Sporn P, Fritsch A (1981) Metabolic disorders in severe abdominal sepsis: glutamine deficiency in skeletal muscle. Clin Nutr 1: 25–41
5. Häussinger D, Lang F (1991) Cell volume in the regulation of hepatic function: a mechanism for metabolic control. Biochim Biophys Acta 1071: 331–350
6. Häussinger D, Roth E, Lang F, Gerok W (1993) Cellular hydration state: an important determinant of protein catabolism in health an disease. Lancet 341: 1330–1332
7. Roth E, Karner J, Ollenschläger G (1990) Glutamin an anabolic effector? J Parent Ent Nutr 14: 130 S–136 S
8. Roth E, Karner J, Roth-Merten A, Winkler S, Valentini L, Schaupp K (1991) Effect of α-ketoglutarate infusions on organ balances of glutamine and glutamate in anaesthetized dogs in the catabolic state. Clin Sci 80: 625–631
9. Lowe DK, Benfell K, Smith RJ, Jacobs DO, Murawsji B, Ziegler TR, Wilmore DW (1990) Safety of glutamine-enriched parenteral nutrient solutions in humans. Am J Clin Nutr 52: 1101–1106
10. Karner J, Roth E, Ollenschläger G, Fürst P, Simmel A, Karner J (1989) Glutamine-containing dipeptides as infusion substrates in the septic state. Surgery 106: 893–900
11. Roth E, Winkler S, Hölzenbein T, Valentini L, Karner J (1992) High load of alanylglutamine in two patients with acute pancreatitis. Clin Nutr 11: 82 S
12. Lowry SF (1993) Anticytokine therapies in sepsis. New Horizons 1: 120–126
13. Werdan K (1993) Neue Aspekte der Sepsis-Behandlung – Additive Therapiemaßnahmen mit Antikörpern und Antagonisten gegen Bakterientoxine

und Sepsismediatoren sowie mit Immunglobulinen. Intensivmedizin 30: 201–217

14. Ziegler EJ, Fisher CF, Sprung CL, Straube RC, Sadoff JC, Foulke GE, Wortel CH, Fink MP, Dellinger RP, Teng NNH, Allen IE, Berrger HJ, Knatterud GL, LoBuglio AF, Smith CR, HA-1A Sepsis Study group (1991) Treatment of gram-negative bacteremia and septic shock with HA-1A human monoclonal antibody against endotoxin – A randomized, double-blind, placebo-controlled trial. N Engl J Med 324: 429–436

15. Greenman RL, Schein RMH, Martin MA, Wenzel RP, MacIntyre NR, Emmanuel G, Chmel H, Kohler RB, McCarthy M, Plouffe J, Russell JA, XOMA Sepsis Study Group (1991) A controlled clinical trial of E5 murine monoclonal IgM antibody to endotoxin in the treatment of gram-negative sepsis. JAMA 266: 1097–1102

16. Engelmann H, Novick D, Wallach D (1990) Two tumor necrosis factor-binding proteins purified from human urine. J Biol Chem 265: 1531–1536

17. Tracey KJ, Fong Y, Hesse DG, Manogue KR, Lee AT, Kuo GC, Lowry SF, Cerami A (1987) Anti-cachectin/TNF monoclonal antibodies prevent septic shock during lethal bacteraemia. Nature 330: 662–664

18. Epstein FH (1993) The role of interleukin-1 in disease. N Engl J Med 328: 106–113

19. Gershenwald JE, Fong YM, Fahey TJ III, et al (1990) Interleukin 1 receptor blockade attenuates the host inflammatory response. Proc Natl Acad Sci USA 87: 4966–70

20. Fisher CJ, Slotman GJ, Opal S (1991) Interleukine-1 receptor antagonist (IL-1ra) reduces mortality in patients with sepsis syndrome. Annual Meeting of the American College of Chest Physicans, San Francisco (Abstract)

21. Fisher C, Dhainaut JF, Pribble J, Knaus W, IL-1ra Phase III Sepsis Syndrome Study Group (1993) Interleukine-1 receptor antagonist: pharmacological and clinical review. International Conference on Sepsis in the ICU: A Masterclass Symposium, London (Abstract)

22. Liljedahl SO, Gemzell CA, Plantin LO, Birke G (1961) Effect of human growth hormone in patients with severe burns. Acta Chir Scand 122: 1–14

23. Ziegler TR, Young LS, Manson JM, Wilmore DW (1988) Metabolic effects of recombinant human growth hormone in patients receiving parenteral nutrition. Ann Surg 208: 6–16

24. Jiang ZM, He GZ, Zhang SY, Wilmore DW (1989) Low-dose growth hormone and hypocaloric nutrition attenuate the protein-catabolic response after major operation. Surgery 210: 513–524

25. Gottardis M, Benzer A, Koller W, Luger TJ, Puhringer F, Hackl J (1991) Improvement of septic syndrome after administration of recombinant human growth hormone (rhGH)? J Trauma 31: 81–86

26. Belcher HJCR, Mercer D, Judkins KC, et al (1991) Biosynthetic human growth hormone in burned patients: a pilot study. Burns 15: 99–107

27. Roth E, Valentini L, Semsroth M, Hölzenbein T, Plattner H, Winkler S, Blum WF, Ranke MB, Hammerle A, Karner J (1992) No nitrogen sparing

effect of recombinant human growth hormone in patients with multiple trauma. J Endocrinol Invest 15: 97 S

28. Voerman HJ, Strack van Schijndel RJM, Groeneveld ABJ, DeBoer H, Nauta JP, van derVeen EA, Thijs LG (1992) Effects of recombinant human growth hormone in patients with severe sepsis. Surgery 216: 648–655

29. Ross R, Miell J, Freeman E, Jones J, Matthews D, Preece M, Buchanan C (1991) Critically ill patients have high basal growth hormone levels with attenuated oscillatory activity associated with low levels of insulin-like growth factor I. Clin Endocrinol 35: 47–54

30. Miell JP, Taylor AM, Jones J, et al (1992) Administration of human recombinant insulin-like growth factor I to patients following major gastrointestinal surgery. Clin Endocrinol 37: 542–551

31. Mauras N, Horber FF, Haymond MW (1992) Low dose recombinant human insulin-like growth factor-I fails to affect protein anabolism but inhibits islet cell secretion in humans. J Clin End Met 75: 1192–1197

32. Roth E, Valentini L, Hölzenbein T, Winkler S, Sautner T, Hörtnagl H, Karner J (1993) Acute effects of insulin-like growth factor I on interorgan amino acid flux in protein-catabolic dogs. Biochem J 296: 765–769

33. Moncada S, Palmer RMJ, Higgs EA (1991) Nitric oxide: physiology, pathophysiology and pharmacology. Pharmacol Rev 43: 109–141

34. Palmer RM (1993) The discovery of nitric oxide in the vessel wall. A unifying concept in the pathogenesis of sepsis. Arch Surg 128: 396–401

35. Lorente JA, Landin L, dePablo P, Renes E, Liste D (1993) L-arginine pathway in the sepsis syndrome. Crit Care Med 21: 1287–1295

36. Roth E, Steininger R, Winkler S, Längle F, Grünberger T, Függer R, Mühlbacher F (1994) – L-Arginine deficiency after liver transplantation as an effect of arginase efflux from the graft. Influence on nitric oxide metabolism. Transplantation 57: 1–6

37. Boeckstegers P, Weidenhöfer ST, Pilz G, Werdan K (1991) Peripheral oxygen availability within skeletal muscle in sepsis and septic shock: comparison to limited infection and cardiogenic shock. Infection 19: 317–323

38. Ochoa JB, Udekwu AO, Billiar TR, Curran RD, Cerra FB, Simmons RL, Peitzman AB (1991) Nitrogen oxide levels in patients after trauma and during sepsis. Ann Surg 214: 621–626

39. Curran RD, Billiar TR, Stuehr DJ, Ochoa JB, Harbrecht BG, Flint SG, Simmons RL (1990) Multiple cytokines are required to induce hepatocyte nitric oxide production and inhibit total protein synthesis. Ann Surg 212: 462–471

40. Geng Y-J, Hansson GK, Holme E (1992) Interferon-gamma and tumor necrosis factor synergize to induce nitric oxide production and inhibit mitochondrial respiration in vascular smooth muscle cells. Circ Res 71: 1268–1276

Korrespondenz: Prof. Dr. E. Roth, Klinik für Chirurgie, Forschungslaboratorien, Währinger Gürtel 18–20, A-1090 Wien, Österreich

Hirnstoffwechsel des Patienten mit Schädel-Hirn-Trauma

C. K. Spiss, W. Schramm und U. M. Illievich

Arbeitsgruppe für Neuroanästhesie und Intensivmedizin, Klinik für Anästhesie und Allgemeine Intensivmedizin, AKH / Universitätskliniken, Wien, Österreich

Einleitung

Das Schädel-Hirn-Trauma (SHT) stellt in Europa und Nordamerika nach wie vor die Hauptursache für Tod oder schwere Behinderung in der Altersgruppe bis 45 Jahre dar [1]. In Österreich erleiden pro Jahr ca. 1400 Menschen ein SHT. 10 % der Unfallopfer versterben bereits am Unfallort, ungefähr 60 % weisen zusätzliche Verletzungen auf. Bei diesen polytraumatisierten Patienten kommt es auf Grund des Blutverlustes, der Hyperkapnie und Hypoxie zu einer Aggravierung der cerebralen Symptomatik.

Pathophysiologie und Pathogenese

Pathogenetisch unterscheiden wir eine primäre und eine sekundäre Hirnschädigung. Die primäre Hirnschädigung tritt in Sekundenbruchteilen aufgrund der direkten Gewalteinwirkung und dem davon getriggerten biochemischen Effekt auf. Als Folge der diffusen axonalen Schädigung [2], die auch Glia- und Endothelzellen inkludiert, kommt es zu einer Störung der Ionenhomöostase mit intrazellulärer Kalziumanreicherung. Daneben bedingen eine intra- und extrazelluläre Azidose, traumatische Mikroblutungen, das Aufbrechen der Blut-Hirnschranke

(BHS) und die eintretende Vasodilatation das Auftreten einer sekundären Hirnschädigung.

Jede Form des ZNS Traumas birgt die Gefahr der fokalen und oder globalen cerebralen Ischämie. Der Ablauf einer bereits aktivierten Mediatorkaskade wird durch die Ischämie aufrechterhalten. Der Zusammenbruch der Kalzium-Homöostase im Sinne eines vermehrten Kalzium Einstroms in die Zelle ist beim ischämischen Zelluntergang von zentraler Bedeutung. Neben dem Versagen der Ionenpumpen im Rahmen des „energy failures" kommt es zur Freisetzung von Neurotransmittern [3], Kininen [4], Arachnoidonsäure [5], Sauerstoffradikalen [6]. und exzitatorischen Aminosäuren. Glutamat, ein excitatorischer Neurotransmitter, wirkt an einer Reihe von Rezeptoren und kann in entsprechender Konzentration *in vitro* [7]. und *in vivo* [8]. zum neuronalen Zelluntergang führen. Glutamat ist nicht nur am Na^+ und Wasser Einstrom, und damit an der akuten Zellschwellung im Rahmen der Ischämie beteiligt, sondern bewirkt sowohl direkt über ionotrope, als auch indirekt mittels second messenger über den metabotropen Rezeptor, einen in der Folge deletären Kalziumeinstrom. Ausgelöst durch die ischämische Depolarisation der Zelle öffnen sich zusätzlich „voltage sensitive" Kalzium Kanäle. Die Akkumulation von intrazellulärem Kalzium bewirkt nun eine Reihe von Prozessen die schließlich zu einer irreversiblen Schädigung der Zelle führen.

Freie Radikale, das heißt Teilchen mit ungepaartem Elektron, die auch unter physiologischen Bedingungen im Intermediärstoffwechsel entstehen werden normalerweise durch natürliche Antioxidantien wie z. B. Tocopherol, Ascorbinsäure, Glutathion, oder Carotine neutralisiert. Auf Grund des Traumas und der Ischämie kommt es zu einem vermehrten Anfall von freien Radikalen [9]. z. B. durch Aktivierung von Cyclooxygenasen und dem vermehrten Abbau der Arachidonsäure. Superoxyd Anionen werden durch die Superoxyd Dismutase in den Mitochondrien zu Wasserstoffperoxid übergeführt. Wasserstoffperoxid, selbst kein Radikal verhält sich aber auf Grund seiner hohen Reaktionsbereitschaft selbst wie ein Radikal. Außerdem wird durch eine von Metallionen (Fe^+, Cu^+) katalysierte Reaktion [10]. die unter physiologischen Bedingungen langsam ablaufende Bildung des toxischen Hydroxylradikals beschleunigt.

Diese entstehenden freien Radikale reagieren mit Wasserstoffatomen aus dem Lipidanteil der Zellmembran und bewirken so eine Öffnung der Zellmembran.

Die Lipidperoxidation verstärkt Zellschädigung und Gefäßpermeabilität [11], Thrombozytenaggregation und die NO-Freisetzung [12]. aus Endothelzellen beeinflussen den weiteren Verlauf zusätzlich ungünstig.

Das klinische Korrelat des Ablaufes dieser Mediatorkaskade ist das Auftreten und in der Folge die Verstärkung eines zytotoxisch-vasogenen Hirnödems sowie eine schwere Störung der cerebralen Autoregulation.

Die irreversible Hirnschädigung tritt dann ein, wenn der cerebrale Blutfluß (CBF) im Mißverhältnis zum metabolischen Bedarf steht. Die Inbalance des cerebralen Sauerstoff Angebot-Bedarfsverhältnisses in Kombination mit der beeinträchtigten Autoregulation der Hirngefäße und des gestörten BHS stellt eine therapeutische Herausforderung dar, der wir uns auf Grund des derzeit verfügbaren Monitorings (z. B. Computertomographie, intracranielle Druckmessung, Transcranielle Dopplersonographie, Bulbusoxymetrie, elektrophysiologisches Monitoring) stellen können.

Hirnödem

Das traumatische Hirnödem ist eine Kombination aus einem vasogenem und zytotoxischem Ödem. Das proteinreiche *interstitielle vasogene* Hirnödem entsteht durch die Schädigung der BHS. Das *intrazelluläre zytotoxische* Hirnödem entwickelt sich auf Grund des Zusammenbruches der Ionenpumpe.

Das *extrazelluläre hydrostatische* Hirnödem hingegen kann perioperativ durch plötzliche Entleerung eines intracraniellen Hämatoms (epidural, subdural, oder intracerebral) als Folge des hydrostatischen Druckgradienten zwischen intra- und extravaskulärem Raum entstehen [13].

Cerebraler Blutfluß

Die unter physiologischen Bedingungen vorhandene Koppelung von cerebralem Blutfluß (CBF) und cerebralem Stoffwechsel

(CMR) [14]. kann nach Trauma gestört sein [15]. Die Folge dieser Entkoppelung kann ein Mißverhältnis zwischen Substratangebot und -nachfrage sein. Besonders bei jungen Patienten bedingt das Trauma ein Stunden bis Tage dauernde hyperämische Phase mit einer Vermehrung des intracraniellen Volumens. Diese Volumsbelastung kann, durch die im knöchernen Schädel nur begrenzte vorhandene Expansionsmöglichkeit, nach Aufbrauchen der cerebralen Reserve(Liquor)räume zu einem intracraniellen Druckanstieg führen. Die Folge davon sind fokale oder schließlich globale Ischämien.

Die unter normalen Verhältnissen vorhandene Autoregulation sichert einen konstanten cerebralen Blutfluß von 50 ml · 100 g Gewebe^{-1} · min^{-1} trotz Änderungen des systemischen Blutdruckes (MAP von 60 bis 130 mm Hg). Auf Grund der im Rahmen eines Traumas auftretenden Störung der Autoregulation wird der CBF druckpassiv, d. h. es besteht eine direkte Abhängigkeit vom mittleren arteriellen Systemdruck und damit vor allem beim schockierten Patienten die Gefahr einer cerebralen Hypoperfusion. Ob eine ausreichende *globale* Hirndurchblutung vorliegt kann mit Hilfe der Bulbusoxymetrie und Bulbuslaktatmessung evaluiert werden [16].

Neben der Beeinträchtigung der Autoregulation besteht beim SHT auch eine schwere Beeinträchtigung der CO_2-Gefäßreagibilität. Im gesunden Gehirn bewirkt Hypokapnie cerebrale Vasokonstriktion und Hyperkapnie cerebrale Vasodilatation. Eine Änderung des pa CO_2 um 1 mm Hg bewirkt eine proportionale Änderung des CBF um 2 ml · 100 g Gewebe^{-1} · min^{-1}. Im Rahmen einer Vasomotorenparalyse kann nun Blut von geschädigten zu normalen Arealen hin geshuntet werden („intracerebral steal"). Die transcranielle Doppler-Sonographie erlaubt nicht nur eine Überprüfung der Gefäßreagibilität, sondern auch eine nicht invasive kontinuierliche Bestimmung der Gehirnperfusion [17].

Endokrine Veränderungen

Ein schweres Trauma verursacht komplexe humorale Veränderungen, welche das sympathische Nervensystem, die hypothalamisch-hypophysäre Achse, die Nebenniere, die Schilddrüse als auch den endokrinen Anteil des Pankreas inkludiert [18].

Der Diabetes Insipidus stellt die wichtigste endokrine Abnormalität dieses Patientenkollektivs dar. Die Ursache liegt in der mehrfachen Schädigung der komplexen Synthese dieses aus 9 Aminosäuren bestehenden hypothalamischen Hormons. Der Gefahr der Hyperosmolarität kann nur durch repetitive Bestimmungen von Natrium im Serum und Harn und adäquater Flüssigkeits-, Elektrolyt- und Hormon substitution begegnet werden.

Durch die gestörte Funktion des Hypothalamus kann es aber auch zu einem Anstieg von ACTH, STH und β Endorphinen kommen. Von klinischer Bedeutung ist jedoch die inadäquat *(hohe)* ADH Sezernierung. Bei ungefähr einem Drittel der Patientin tritt dieses Syndrom der vermehrten ADH Ausschüttung (SIADH) [19] zutage. Die Folge davon ist eine Flüssigkeitsretention mit einer Verdünnungshyponatriämie und Gefahr des hypoosmolaren Hirnödems.

Auf Grund des erhöhten ACTH-Spiegels steigen die Plasmacortisolspiegel nach Trauma auf ein Vielfaches der Normalwerte an. Ein Zusammenhang zwischen Plasmacortisolspiegel und der Komadauer wurde von Steinbok et al. nachgewiesen [20].

Glukosestoffwechsel

Bei einer Vielzahl von Patienten besteht in der akuten Phase nach SHT bereits eine Hyperglykämie. Die Ursache für diese Hyperglykämie ist die durch das Trauma bedingte sympathoadrenerge Aktivität mit erhöhten ACTH- und Plasmacortisolspiegeln.

Die Beobachtung, daß erhöhte Blutzuckerspiegel einen negativen Einfluß auf die ischämiebedingte Nervenzellschädigung haben, konnte in einer Vielzahl von experimentellen Untersuchungen [21, 22], als auch bei Patienten mit Schädel-Hirn-Traumen nachgewiesen werden [23]. Die Ursache für die zusätzliche neuronale Schädigung scheint in der durch die anaerobe Glykolyse bedingten vermehrten Laktatansammlung mit intrazellulärer Azidose zu liegen. Obwohl eine vermehrte Laktat-

ansammlung tierexperimentell nachgewiesen wurde [24], kann
Laktat *per se* nicht als Verursacher der neuronalen Schädigung
bezeichnet werden. Trotz ungeklärter Genese der hyper-
glycämischen neuronalen Schädigung im Rahmen eines SHT
muß eine weitere iatrogene Anhebung des Blutzuckerspiegels –
sei es direkt (Glukosegabe), oder indirekt (Cortisongabe) – unbedingt vermieden werden [25].

Literatur

1. Kraus JF (1993) Epidemiology of head injury. In: Cooper PR (ed) Wil-
    liams & Wilkins, New York, pp 1–25
2. Adams JH, Graham DI, Doyle D (1984) Diffuse axonal injury in head
    injuries caused by a fall. Lancet 22: 1420–1422
3. Faden AI, Demediuk P, Panter SS (1989) The role of excitatory amino
    acids and NMDA receptors in traumatic brain injury. Science 244: 789–800
4. Maier HK, Baethmann AJ, Lange M, et al (1984) The kallikrein-kinin sy-
    stem as mediator in vasogenic brain edema, part 2. Studies on kinin for-
    mation in focal and perifocal brain tissue. J Neurosurg 61: 97–106
5. Papadopoulos S, Black KL, Hoff JD (1989) Cerebral edema induced by
    arachidonic acid: role of leucocytes and 5-lipoxygenase products. Neu-
    rosurgery 25: 369–372
6. Ikeda Y, Long DM (1990) The molecular basis of brain injury and brain
    edema: the role of oxygen free radicals. Neurosurgery 27: 1–11
7. Choi DW, Koh JY, Peters S (1988) Pharmacology of glutamate neu-
    rotoxicity in cortical cell culture: attenuation by NMDA antagonists.
    J Neurosci 8: 185–196
8. Benveniste H, Jørgensen MB, Sandberg M, et al (1989) Ischemic damage in
    hippocampal CA1 is dependent on glutamate release and intact innervation
    from CA3. J Cereb Blood Flow Metab 9: 629–639
9. Lundgren J, Zhang H, Agardh CD, et al (1991) Acidosis-induced ischemic
    brain damage: are free radicals involved? J Cereb Blood Flow Metab 11:
    587–596
10. Halliwell B, Gutteridge JM (1985) The importance of free radicals and
    catalytic metal ions in human diseases. Mol Aspects Med 8: 89–193
11. Moore WS, Hall AD (1968) Ulcerated atheroma of the carotid artery.
    A cause of transient cerebral ischemia. Am J Surg 116: 237–242
12. Nowicki JP, Duval D, Poignet H, et al (1991) Nitric oxide mediates neu-
    ronal death after focal cerebral ischemia in the mouse. Eur J Pharmacol
    204: 339–340
13. Baker RN, Broward JA, Fang HC, et al (1966) Anticoagulant therapy of
    cerebral infarction: report of a national cooperative study. Res Publ Assoc
    Res Nerv Ment Dis 41: 287–302

14. Siesjo BK (1984) Cerebral circulation and metabolism. J Neurosurg 60: 883–908
15. Obrist WD, Langfitt TW, Jaggi JL (1984) Cerebral blood flow and metabolism in comatose patients with acute head injury. Relationship to intracranial hypertension. J Neurosurg 61: 241
16. Dearden NM (1991) Jugular bulb venous oxygen saturation in the management of the severe head injury. Curr Opin Anaesth 4: 279–286
17. Newell DW (1992) Transcraniell Doppler: clinical and experimental uses. Cerebrovasc Brain Met Rev 4: 122–143
18. Woolf PD (1992) Hormonal responses to trauma. Crit Care Med 20: 216–226
19. Born JD, Hans P, Smitz S, et al (1985) Syndrom of inappropriate secretion of antiduretic hormone after severe head injury. Surg Neurol 23: 283–287
20. Steinbok, P, Thompson G (1979) Serum cortisol abnormalities after cranial cerebral trauma. Neurosurgery 5: 559–565
21. Lanier WL, Stangland KJ, Scheithauer BW, et al (1987) The effects of dextrose infusion and head position on neurologic outcome after complete cerebral ischemia in primates: examination of a model. Anesthesiology 66: 39–48
22. Kraft SA, Larson CP, Shuer LM, et al (1990) Effect of hyperglycemia on neuronal changes in a rabbit model of focal cerebral ischemia. Stroke 21: 447–450
23. Lam AM, Winn RH, Cullen BF, et al (1991) Hyperglycemia and neurological outcome in patients with head injury. J Neurosurg 75: 545–551
24. Hoffman WE, Braucher E, Pelligrino DA, et al (1990) Brain lactate and neurologic outcome following incomplete ischemia in fasted, nonfasted, and glucose-loaded rats. Anesthesiology 72: 1045–1050
25. Sieber FE, Traystman RJ (1992) Special issues: glucose and the brain. Crit Care Med 20: 104–114

Korrespondenz: Prof. Dr. C. K. Spiss, Klinik für Anästhesie und Allgemeine Intensivmedizin, Universität Wien, Währinger Gürtel 18–20, A-1090 Wien, Österreich

Zellstoffwechsel des Alveolarepithels Typ II: Bedeutung bei der Therapie des ARDS

W. Schobersberger, F. Friedrich und G. Putz

Klinik für Anästhesie und Allgemeine Intensivmedizin,
Universität Innsbruck, Österreich

Einleitung

Das ARDS („adult respiratory distress syndrome") wurde erstmals 1967 von Ashbaugh und Mitarbeitern [1]. beschrieben. Trotz der vielschichtigen Ursachen wie u. a. Sepsis, Schock, Pneumonie, Trauma und Aspiration ist das ARDS unabhängig von der Ätiologie gekennzeichnet durch a) eine ausgeprägte, Sauerstoff-refraktäre arterielle Hypoxämie, b) einen erhöhten intrapulmonalen Shunt, c) eine verminderte Lungencompliance und d) ein reduziertes Lungenvolumen bei fehlendem Hinweis auf linksventrikuläres Versagen.

Bezüglich einer ausführlichen Darstellung der Pathophysiologie des ARDS sei auf die mannigfaltige Literatur verwiesen [2, 3]. Die pathophysiologische Sequenz der Ereignisse, die das ARDS zur Folge hat, ist noch nicht restlos geklärt. Gemeinsame Endstrecke der verschiedenen ARDS-induzierenden Noxen ist ein Schaden im Bereich der Alveolen, der letztendlich die Integrität der alveolocapillären Membran beeinträchtigt. Folge ist das Lungenödem, alveolär wie interstitiell, als typisches klinisches Zeichen des ARDS in der Frühphase.

Untersuchungen in den letzten Jahren erbrachten Hinweise, daß das ARDS mit einer gestörten Funktion des Lungensurfactants einhergeht. Im folgenden Abschnitt wird auf die Bedeutung des Alveolarepithels hinsichtlich Physiologie und Pathophysiologie des Surfactant-Stoffwechsels näher eingegangen, sowie eine Übersicht über den derzeitigen Wissensstand der Surfactant-Applikation beim ARDS gegeben.

Zusammensetzung des pulmonalen Surfactants

Surfactant ist ein komplexes Gemisch aus Lipiden und Proteinen mit einem geringen Anteil an Kohlehydraten (für Details siehe [4, 5]). Quantitativ stellt die Lipidfraktion mit 85 %–90 % den größten Anteil am Surfactant dar. Hievon sind etwa 90 % ein Gemisch aus Phospholipiden. Als wichtigstes Phospholipid ist das Phosphatidylcholin zu nennen, dessen Anteil am Surfactant etwa 80 % beträgt und das größtenteils als Dipalmitoyl-phosphatidylcholin (DPPC) vorliegt. Infolge der hydrophoben und hydrophilen Eigenschaften ist DPPC maßgeblich an der Verminderung der Oberflächenspannung an der Grenzfläche zwischen Luft und Flüssigkeit beteiligt. Als weitere Surfactant-Phospholipide sind Phosphatidyglycerol (PG), Phosphatidyl-äthanolamin, Phosphatidylinositol und Sphingomyelin zu nennen. Der Gesamt-Proteinanteil am Surfactant beträgt etwa 10 %. Für die Funktion des Surfactants am wichtigsten sind die vier bisher identifizierten Surfactant spezifischen Proteine (SP). SP-A dürfte eine wichtige Rolle in der Ausbildung einer Vorstufe des alveolären Monolyers, dem sog. „tubulären Myelin", spielen. Zusätzlich dürfte dem SP-A über Unterstützung der Aktivität der Alveolar-Makrophagen eine wichtige Funktion im lokalen Abwehrsystem zukommen. SP-A vermag weiters die Konzentration des alveolären Surfactants mitzuregulieren. Es hemmt die Sekretion von Phosphatidylcholin aus kultivierten Typ II Alveolarzellen [6]. und steigert die Aufnahme von Surfactantlipiden in das Alveolarepithel [7, 8]. SP-B und SP-C sind wichtig für die Ausbildung eines funktionstüchtigen Surfactant-Monolayers. Die Bedeutung des SP-D bleibt nach wie vor umstritten.

Änderungen des pulmonalen Surfactants beim ARDS

Chemische und physikalische Analysen der Lavageflüssigkeit von Patienten mit ARDS und von Tieren mit akuter Lungenschädigung erbrachten den Nachweis, daß sowohl quantitative wie qualitative Störungen des Surfactants vorhanden sind: Der Gesamtgehalt an Phospholipid war entweder unverändert oder vermindert, wobei der Anteil an PC bzw. DPPS und PG am Gesamtgehalt der Phospholipide stets reduziert war [9, 10, 11]. Pison und Mitarbeiter [12]. erbrachten ferner den Nachweis, daß die alveoläre Konzentration an SP-A bei polytraumatisierten Patienten mit ARDS signifikant vermindert war. Die Fähigkeit des Surfactants, unter Kompression die Oberflächenspannung zu reduzieren, war in mehreren Untersuchungen eingeschränkt, was sich in einem Anstieg der minimalen Oberflächenspannung zeigte [13].

Mögliche Mechanismen der Surfactant-Dysfunktion beim ARDS

Die pathophysiologischen Vorgänge, die eine Surfactant-Dysfunktion zur Folge haben, sind mannigfaltig. Da Surfactant ausschließlich von den Alveolarepithelzellen Typ II produziert und in die alveoläre Subphase abgegeben wird, ist verständlich, daß Noxen, die diese Zellen direkt schädigen, mit einer Störung im Surfactant-Metabolismus einhergehen.

Eine der Hauptursachen für die Surfactant-Dysfunktion steht im Zusammenhang mit der massiven Flüssigkeitsverschiebung von capillär nach alveolär und der damit verbundenen Proteinansammlung im Alveolarraum während der Frühphase des ARDS. Nebst der auftretenden Gasaustauschstörung durch das eiweißreiche Lungenödem, besitzen gewisse Proteine der Ödemflüssigkeit, wie Fibrinogen, Fibrinmonomere, Albumin und Hämoglobin [14], sowie das C-reaktive Protein [15]. die Potenz, Surfactant zu inaktivieren. Hyperoxie, deren klinische Anwendung häufig im Rahmen des ARDS notwendig ist, kann ebenfalls eine diffuse Schädigung des Alveolarepithels bewirken und die Phospholipid-Biosynthese des Surfactants vermindern [16]. Auch die Phospholipase A2, ein Enzym, das wahrscheinlich am ARDS infolge Pancreatitis oder Sepsis mitbeteiligt ist, vermag Phospholipide des Surfactants abzubauen [17]. Weiters ist bekannt, daß E. coli-Endotoxin die Surfactant-Synthese beeinträchtigt [18].

Grundüberlegungen zu Surfactant-Applikationen bei Patienten mit ARDS

Exogen zugeführter Surfactant wird in der Neonatologie beim IRDS („infant respiratory distress syndrome") bereits seit mehreren Jahren erfolgreich eingesetzt. Welche positiven Effekte könnte man aufgrund dieser Erfahrungen der Surfactant-Applikation beim ARDS erwarten?

Im Vordergrund der erwarteten Wirkungen steht der Einfluß von Surfactant auf die Lungenmechanik:

a) Während tiefer Inspiration adsorbiert Surfactant rasch an die Grenzschicht Luft-Wasser und bedingt, daß die Oberflächenspannung in der Lunge möglichst wenig über den Äquilibriumwert von 25 mN/m steigt. Der Anteil der Oberflächenkräfte an dem durch Einatmung erzeugten Retraktionsdruck bleibt somit klein; die Atemarbeit wird folgedessen minimiert.

b) Während der durch die Exspiration hervorgerufenen Kompression des adsorbierten Films wird die Oberflächenspannung auf Werte gegen 0 mN/m erniedrigt. Dadurch wird der Anteil kontraktiler Kräfte so weit verringert, daß sich die Lunge am Beginn der Einatmung schon bei einer kleinen Druckdifferenz zu entfalten beginnt.

c) Der Film soll am Ende der Ausatmung unter dem Druck, der auf ihm lastet, nicht kollabieren. Auf diese Art und Weise kann die Oberflächenspannung während Ruheatmung über längere Zeit weit unterhalb des Äquilibriumwertes bleiben, womit einem Kollaps der Lunge wirkungsvoll vorgebeugt wird.

Als weitere mögliche Vorteile der Surfactant-Gabe werden ein verbessertes Ventilations-Perfusions-Verhältnis und eine Verminderung des pulmonalen Shuntvolumens diskutiert. Letztendlich sollte der pulmonale Gasaustausch verbessert werden. Als klinisch-therapeutische Konsequenz sollte das aggressive Beatmungsregime vermindert werden können (Reduktion der inspiratorischen O_2-Konzentration, des inspiratorischen Spitzendrucks, des PEEP-Niveaus u. a.). Das Herzminutenvolumen und der O_2-Transport soll verbessert sowie die Möglichkeit eines Barotraumas des Lungenparenchyms durch die Vermeidung hoher Atemwegsdrücke und intrathorakaler

Drücke minimiert werden. Durch die Verbesserung der Integrität des Alveolarepithels soll infolge weniger Lecks der Flüssigkeitsaustritt in den Alveolarraum reduziert und das Auftreten potenter Inhibitoren des Surfactants (siehe oben) verringert werden. Somit könnte letztendlich das Auftreten hyaliner Membranen im Alveolarraum als Spätfolge des ARDS eingeschränkt werden.

Durch die Kenntnis von Struktur und Funktion der meisten Komponenten des menschlichen Surfactants werden diverse Produkte für den klinischen Einsatz angeboten, die in ihrer Zusammensetzung dem natürlichen Surfactant in der Lunge ähnlich sind (Tabelle 1, mod. nach [3]). „Natürlicher Surfactant" aus humaner Amnionflüssigkeit steht infolge der geringen Menge für den routinemäßigen klinischen Gebrauch nicht zur Verfügung. Am häufigsten werden klinisch die „modifizierten natürlichen Surfactants" verwendet wie Survanta (= Surfactant-TA), Alveofact oder Curosurf. Zur Produktgruppe der „künstlichen Surfactantpräparate", die in vitro synthetisiert werden, zählen Exo-

Tabelle 1

	Quelle	Komponenten	Beispiele
Natürlicher Surfactant	Menschliche oder tierische Alveolar-Lavage Flüssigkeit, Amnion-Flüssigkeit	Phospholipide, Neutrale Lipide, Proteine	Helsinki, San Diego
Modifizierter natürlicher Surfactant	Menschliche oder tierische Alveolar-Lavage Flüssigkeit, Lungenextract	Phospholipide, Neutrale Lipide, Proteine	Surfactant-TA, Curosurf, CLSE
Künstlicher Surfactant	In-Vitro Synthese	DPPC ± ein Alkohol	Exosurf, ALEC
Synthetischer natürlicher Surfactant	In-Vitro-Synthese	Phospholipide, Neutrale Lipide, Surfactant-spezifische Apoproteine, (SP-A, SP-B, SP-C)	California Biotechnology (nicht im klinischen Einsatz)

surf und ALEC. Surfactants die synthetische Peptide oder rekombinante Proteine enthalten, dürften in absehbarer Zeit für die klinische Anwendung im Handel verfügbar sein.

Klinische Erfahrungen mit der Applikation von exogenem Surfactant

Untersuchungen über die Surfactant-Therapie beim ARDS in der Humanmedizin beschränken sich in der Literatur fast ausschließlich auf Kasuistiken. Lachmann [19] beschrieb die Anwendung von natürlichen Surfactant-Phospholipiden in einer Dosis von 300 mg/kg KG via tracheale Instillation bei einem Patienten mit Sepsis und schwerem ARDS. Es wurde hierbei eine transiente Verbesserung des Gasaustausches beobachtet. In einer Kasuistik von Nosaka und Mitarbeiter [20] wurde Surfactant-TA zwei Erwachsenen appliziert. Eine Patientin mit schwersten Verbrennungen erhielt Surfactant in einer Dosis von täglich 240 mg 15 mal in einem Zeitraum von 38 Tagen und einem Patienten mit postoperativer Pneumonie wurde dieselbe Dosis 3 mal verabreicht. Die berichteten Verbesserungen im Gasaustausch und im Thoraxröntgen waren trotz der niedrigen Dosierung erstaunlich. Stubbig und Mitarbeiter [21] berichten über die endobronchiale Applikation von 38 mg/kg KG Surfactantsuspension (Alveofact) bei einem jungen Mann nach schwerem Thoraxtrauma. Nach initialer Verschlechterung des Gasaustausches vermutlich aufgrund endobronchialer Krusten unbekannter Genese kam es nach 24 Stunden zu einer deutlichen Verbesserung der Lungenfunktion (Verringerung des inspiratorischen O_2-Anteils und des PEEP-Niveaus). Spragg und Mitarbeiter [3] beschrieben die Auswirkungen der Instillation von 50 mg/kg KG Curosurf bei 6 Patienten mit ARDS. Während bei 4 Patienten eine transiente Verbesserung des Gasaustausches festgestellt wurde und ein Patient sogar eine deutliche permanente Verbesserung zeigte, war diese Therapie bei nur einem Patienten ohne Erfolg geblieben.

Kürzlich haben wir uns zur Applikation von Surfactant bei einem 32jährigen Patienten mit akutem Lungenversagen bei CMV-Pneumonie und Z.n. Nierentransplantation 2 Monate zuvor entschieden. Infolge massiver Verschlechterung des pulmonalen Gasaustausches trotz zunehmender Beatmungsinvasivität wurde zunächst mit der extrakorporalen Membranoxygenierung (ECMO) begonnen. Unter ECMO normalisierten sich die arteriellen Blutgaswerte. Nach 7 Tagen unter ECMO wurde mit dem Entwöhnen begonnen. Die Beatmung zu diesem Zeitpunkt bestand aus BIPAP-Beatmung (oberes Druckniveau 20 cmH_2O, unteres Druckniveau 11 cmH_2O, Verhältnis Inspiration : Expiration = 1 : 2, FIO_2 0,5) bei zusätzlicher Spontanatmung (Atemfrequenz um 11/min.; Atemminutenvolumen ca. 2 l/min). Um den „Weaning"-Prozeß von der ECMO bei einer möglicherweise noch bestehenden Surfactant-Dysfunktion zu beschleunigen, wurde mit der Surfactant-Applikation begonnen. Der Patient erhielt insgesamt 8 mg Curosurf (200 mg/kg bei geschätztem KG von 40 kg) fiberoptisch in 5 Portionen zu je 20 ml in die einzelnen Lappenbronchien instilliert. Für die Dauer des Applikationsvorganges wurde der Patient relaxiert und bei 100 % O_2 mit CPAP bei gleichzeitiger Erhöhung des Oxygenatorflusses beatmet. Die Surfactant-Applikation ließ sich problemlos durchführen. Anschließend wurde der Patient mit BIPAP bei gleicher Respiratoreinstellung wie vor Surfactantgabe weiterbeatmet. Das Thoraxröntgen zeigte 1 Stunde nach Surfactant-Applikation im Vergleich zum Röntgenbild vor Therapiebeginn keine Änderungen. Im 7 Stunden nach Surfactant-Therapie angefertigten Thoraxröntgen fanden sich jedoch über beiden Lungen deutliche Aufhellungen. Die Compliance blieb unverändert, die FIO_2 und der Frischgasfluß der ECMO konnten in den nächsten beiden Tagen deutlich reduziert werden. Vier Tage nach Surfactant-Applikation verstarb jedoch der Patient an einem Kreislaufversagen im Rahmen eines septischen Schocks.

Infolge der bislang nur spärlichen klinischen Berichte bleiben noch zahlreiche Fragen bezüglich exogener Surfactant-Applikation beim ARDS offen:

Indikationsstellung, Therapiebeginn: Es ist derzeit nicht bekannt, ob sich, vom ätiologischen Standpunkt aus, alle Formen des ARDS in gleicher Weise für eine Surfactant-Therapie eignen. Nicht unwesentlich für den Erfolg der Therapie ist der Zeitpunkt des Therapiebeginns mit Surfactant. Exogen zugeführter Surfactant kann nur vorübergehend die endogene Surfactant-Dysfunktion ersetzen. Eine rechtzeitige Surfactant-Applikation vor Ausschöpfung des Beatmungsregimes scheint uns vordergründig, um die mit zunehmenden Umbauprozessen im Alveolarepithel einhergehende Defektheilung mit Ausbildung hyaliner Membranen zu begrenzen.

Applikation: Die Verabreichung von Surfactant über ein fiberoptisches Bronchoskop hat den Vorteil, daß fraktionierte Dosen unter Sicht in verschiedene Lungenareale appliziert werden können. Ob Surfactant adäquat über einen Vernebler verabreicht werden kann, wird derzeit untersucht. Zumindest tierexperimentell sind diesbezügliche Therapieerfolge beim ARDS beschrieben [22].

Dosis: Nimmt man die Dosierungen aus der Neonatologie in Abhängigkeit vom Präparat mit 50 bis 200 mg/kg KG, so beträgt die Einzeldosis an Surfactant in Abhängigkeit vom Präparat 3,5 g bis 14 g für einen 70 kg schweren Erwachsenen. Die Frage nach der optimalen Dosis ist aber noch offen. Weiters ungeklärt ist auch die Frage, über welchen Zeitraum repetitive Dosen von Surfactant sinnvoll sind.

Kosten: Limitierend sind nicht zuletzt die enormen Kosten der Surfactant-Therapie, die für eine einmalige Bolusgabe ca. öS 300.000,– und mehr betragen.

Zusammenfassung: Die Therapie des ARDS stellt nach wie vor höchste Anforderungen an den Intensivmediziner. Jeder neue therapeutische Ansatz, der sich rational als Mosaik in das komplexe Bild des ARDS einfügen läßt, ist primär als positiv zu betrachten und genauestens zu untersuchen. Trotz noch ausständiger kontrollierter Studien sehen wir derzeit die Anwendung von exogenem Surfactant inmitten der konventionellen therapeutischen Maßnahmen als vielversprechenden Therapieansatz beim ARDS.

Literatur

1. Absaugh DG, Bigelow DB, Petty TL, Levine BE (1967) Acute respiratory distress in adults. Lancet ii: 319–323
2. Seeger W, Günther A, Walmrath HD, Grimminger F, Lasch HG (1993) Alveolar surfactant and adult respiratory distress syndrome. Clin Invest 71: 177–190
3. Spragg RG, Gilliard N, Richman P, Smith RM, Hite D, Pappert D, Heldt GP, Meritt TA (1992) The adult respiratory distress syndrome: clinical

aspects relevant to surfactant supplementation. In: Robertson B, Van Golde LMG, Batenburg JJ (eds) Pulmonary surfactant: from molecular biology to clinical practice. Elsevier Science Publishers, pp 685–703

4. Hamm H, Fabel H, Bartsch W (1992) The surfactant system of the adult lung: physiology and clinical perspectives. Clin Invest 70: 637–657

5. Hawgood S, Shiffer K (1991) Structure and properties of the surfactant-associated proteins. Ann Rev Physiol 53: 375–394

6. Dobbs LG, Wright JR, Gonzales R, Venstrom K, Nellenbogen J (1987) Pulmonary surfactant and its components inhibit secretion of phosphatidylcholine from cultured rat alevolar type II cells. Proc Natl Acad Sci 84: 1010–1014

7. Tsuzuki A, Kuroki Y, Akino T (1993) Pulmonary surfactant protein A-meditated uptake of phosphatidylcholine by alveolar type II cells. Am Physiol 265 (Lung Cell Mol Physiol 9): L193–L199

8. Wright JR, Wager RE, Hawgood S, Dobbs LG, Clements JA (1987) Surfactant apoprotein Mr = 26.000–36.000 enhances uptake of liposomes by type II cells. J Biol Chem 262: 2888–2894

9. Petty TL, Silvers WG, Paul GW, Stanford RE (1979) Abnormalities in lung elastic properties and surfactant function in adult respiratory distress syndrome. Chest 75: 571–574

10. Hallman M, Spragg RG, Harrell JH, Moser KM, Gluck L (1982) Evidence of lung surfactant abnormality in respiratory failure: study of broncho-alveolar lavage phospholipids, surface activity, phospholipase activity, and plasma myoinositol. J Clin Invest 70: 673–683

11. Pison U, Obertacke U, Brand M, Seeger W, Joka T, Bruch J, Schmidt-Neuerburg KP (1990) Altered pulmonary surfactant in uncomplicated and septicemia-complicated courses of acute respiratory failure. J Trauma 30: 19–26

12. Pison RL, Obertacke U, Seeger W, Hawgood S (1992) Surfactant protein A (SP-A) is decreased in acute parenchymal lung injury associated with polytrauma. Eur J Clin Invest 22: 712–718

13. Greogry TJ, Longmore WJ, Moxley MA, Whitsett JA, Reed CR, Fowler III AA, Hudson LD, Maunder RJ, Crim C, Hyers TM (1991) Surfactant chemical composition and biophysical activity in acute respiratory distress syndrome. J Clin Invest 88: 1976–1981

14. Spragg RG, Richman P, Gilliard N, Merritt TA (1987) The future for surfactant therapy of the adult respiratory distress syndrome. In: Lachmann B (ed) Surfactant replacement therapy. Springer, New York, pp 203–211

15. Li JJ, Sanders RL, McAdam KP, Hales CA, Thompson BT, Gelfand JA, Burke JF (1989) Impact of C-reactive protein (CRP) on surfactant function. J Trauma 29: 1690–1697

16. Holm BA, Matalon S, Finkelstein JN, Notter RH (1988) Type II pneumocyte changes during hyperoxic lung injury and recovery. J Appl Physiol 65: 2672–2678

17. Edelson JD, Vadas P, Villar J, Mullen JBM, Pruzanski W (1991) Acute lung injury induced by phospholipase A2. Am Rev Resp Dis 143: 1102–1109
18. Oldham KT, Guice KS, Stetson PS, Wolfe RR (1989) Bacteremia-induced suppression of alveolar surfactant production. J Surg Res 47: 397–402
19. Lachmann B (1987) Surfactant replacement in acute respiratory failure: animal studies and first clinical trials. In: Lachmann B (ed) Surfactant replacement therapy. Springer, New York, pp 212–223
20. Nosaka S, Sakai T, Yonekura M, Yoshikawa K (1990) Surfactant for adults with respiratory failure. Lancet 336: 947–948
21. Subbig K, Schmidt H, Böhrer H, Huster Th, Bach A, Motsch J (1992) Surfactantapplikation bei akutem Lungenversagen. Anaesthesist 41: 555–558
22. Lewis J, Tabor B, Ikegami M, Jobe A (1991) Physiological response to aerosolized surfactant in lung-lavaged sheep. Am Rev Resp Dis 143: A769

Korrespondenz: Dr. W. Schobersberger, Universitätsklinik für Anästhesie und Allgemeine Intensivmedizin, Universität Innsbruck, Anichstraße 35, A-6020 Innsbruck, Österreich

The effects of routine intensive care interactions on metabolic rate in ventilated patients

Ch. Weissmann

College of Physicians and Surgeons, Columbia University,
New York, NY, U.S.A.

The intensive care unit is a dynamic setting where critically ill patients receive extensive and constant care. They undergo many clinical and nursing interventions as a part of their routine care. These result in changes in oxygen consumption and carbon dioxide production that are accompanied by alterations in the outputs of the cardiovascular and respiratory systems. This provides an opportunity to examine the physiological response of critically ill patients to acute increases in oxygen demand. More practically, oxygen consumption and carbon dioxide production are frequently measured to calculate energy expenditure for use in planning nutritional regimens. The intrinsic state of the patient (sleeping, resting, moving etc) affects the determination of energy expenditure and must be accounted for.

Many routine nursing and physician interactions alter metabolic rate [1]. When making metabolic measurements the intrinsic state of the patients during the measurements must be considered. We have established definitions of various events to permit consistent reporting [1]. Sleeping is defined as a state where the patient was not aroused by surrounding events. Resting is defined as lying motionless with eyes open responsive to surrounding events. A written log is kept of the activity state, sleep, rest or other, of the patient during metabolic measurements. The oxygen consumption and carbon dioxide production values during rest are used to calculate the resting energy expenditure (REE). This reference state is used in the formulation of nutritional support regimens and for intra and interpatient comparisons of metabolic state.

Metabolic rates below resting levels are found during sleep and sedation. Oxygen consumption average about 9 % below resting values during sleep [1]. Sedatives and muscle relaxants can also decrease metabolic rate 10–15 % below resting values. A variety of activities result in increases of metabolic rate of about 10–20 % above resting values. These are routine daily activities that are not painful but involve arousal from the resting state, external stimulation and both active and passive limb movements. Voluntary movements of the patient's bodies and limbs produce increases of similar magnitude in oxygen consumption and carbon dioxide production. These low level activities are associated with variable increases in heart rate, systolic blood pressure, oxygen delivery and oxygen extraction [2]. Chest physical therapy results in increases above resting levels in oxygen consumption of 40–50 % [1, 2]. These are probably due to a variety of factors including pain associated with an increase in catecholamine secretion, movement of the limbs and increased muscular tension in the limbs, chest and abdomen. The weaning of patients from mechanical ventilation results in an increase in metabolic rate likely from anxiety and increased work of breathing [3].

Total energy expenditure

The initial step in designing a nutritional regimen is to assess the patient's caloric needs. This can be done by either measuring or estimating the patient's resting energy expenditure and adding factors for daily activity or by measuring total energy expenditure. The latter is the energy expended in a 24 hour period. The activity factor is thus the difference between resting and total energy expenditure. Ten percent is usually added to the resting energy expenditure for bedridden patients, while 20 % is added for the sedentary individual. In mechanically ventilated patients the acitivity factors have been reported to be 5 to 10 % greater than resting energy expenditure [4]. The duration of activity in these patients tends to be short and they also spend much time sleeping or sedated. In some ICU patients who are heavily sedated total energy expenditure is lower than resting energy expenditure.

Integrative physiology in the critically ill

Critically ill patients often have compromised respiratory and hemodynamic function. Yet, they frequently must respond to the acute increase in oxygen demand. We studied this response using chest physical therapy as the stimulus [5]. To accommodate the average increase in oxygen consumption of 52 %, there was a 35 % increase in tissue oxygen extraction and a 17 % increase in oxygen delivery. Cardiac output also increased while mixed venous oxygen saturation decreased (rest: 72 %, chest physical therapy: 64 %). Heart rate increased significantly (rest: 97 bpm, chest physical therapy: 107 bpm) as did blood pressure (rest: 135/68, chest physical therapy: 155/76). System vascular resistance did not change. Along with the increase in metabolic and hemodynamic parameters, there were increases in minute and alveolar ventilation. Yet these were not high enough to eliminate the increased CO_2 produced, and there were thus small increases in $PaCO_2$. Mathews and Weissman [6] observed that when there were ST segment changes following abdominal aortic surgery they often occurred during chest physical therapy. The responses to this acute increase in oxygen demand is likely the result of an increase in catecholamines caused by discomfort and pain along with an exercise-like response due to limb movement. The type of change from resting levels of oxygen delivery and oxygen extraction caused by chest physical therapy are affected by resting hemodynamic profiles [7].

Many ICU interventions such as chest physiotherapy and wound debridement are discomforting and result in significant responses by the cardiovascular and respiratory systems. It would thus be useful to attenuate these responses during the period of stress without causing any problems once the stimulation had stopped. This requires the use of short acting yet potent analgesics and sedatives. Klein et al. [8] found that   1.5 µg/ kg of fentanyl administered intravenously in mechanically ventilated patients two minutes prior to chest physical therapy had no effect on the increase in oxygen consumption or carbon dioxide elimination, but did attenuates the heart rate response. 3.0 µg/kg of fentanyl attenuated both the blood pressure and heart rate responses. Alfentanil 30 µg/kg and 60 µg/kg had similar effects [9]. Also observed during the alfentanil study was suppression by the drug of minute ventilation, resulting in significant CO_2 retention in some patients. These studies show that moderate doses of fentanyl and alfentanil do not alter metabolic response, but modify the hemodynamic ones, likely as the result of alfentanil and fentanyl's vagotonic properties. Other classes of sedatives and analgesics may better attenuate the responses to ICU interventions.

Summary

Routine ICU care interactions can cause significant alterations in metabolism and cardiopulmonary function. This has ramifications when designing nutritional support regimens and in patients with marginal organ function.

References

1. Weissman C, Kemper M, Damask MC, Askanazi J, Hyman AI, Kinney JM (1983) The effect of routine intensive care interactions on metabolic rate. Med 98: 41–44

2. Weissman C, Kemper M (1991) The oxygen uptake-oxygen delivery relationship during ICU interventions. Chest 99: 430–435

3. Kemper M, Weissman C, Askanazi J, Kinney JM, Hyman AI (1987) Metabolic and respiratory changes during weaning from mechanical ventilation. Chest 92: 979–983

4. Weissman C, Kemper M, Elwyn DH, Askanazi J, Hyman AI, Kinney JM (1986) The energy expenditure of the mechanically ventilated critically ill patient: an analysis. Chest 89: 254–259

5. Weissman C, Kemper M (1993) Stressing the critically ill patient: the cardiopulmonary and metabolic response to an acute increase in oxygen consumption. J Crit Care 8: 100–108

6. Mathews D, Weissman C (1990) Real-time ST segment analysis following abdominal aortic aneurysm reaction. Anesthesiology 73: A 1228

7. Weissman C, Kemper M, Harding J (1992) The response of critically ill patients to acute increases in oxygen demand: hemodynamic subsets. Crit Care Med 20: S 113

8. Klein P, Kemper M, Weissman C, Rosenbaum SH, Askanazi J, Hyman AI (1988) Attenuation of the hemodynamic responses to chest physical therapy. Chest 93: 38–42
9. Harding J, Kemper M, Weissman C (1993) Alfentanil attenuates the cardiopulmonary response of critically ill patients to an acute increase in oxygen demand. Anesth Analg (in press)
10. Cohen D, Kemper MC, Weissman C (1993) Attenuation in increases in metabolic and cardiopulmonary demand by propofol (abstract). Anesthesiology (in press)

Correspondence: Ch. Weissman, MD, Professor of Anesthesiology and Medicine, College of Physicians and Surgeons, Columbia University, New York, NY 10032, U.S.A.

Gibt es eine spezielle Ernährung für den Patienten mit respiratorischer Insuffizienz?

W. Höltermann, P. Lukasewitz, N. Lemcke, L. Leuchter und
M. van Wickern

Abteilung für Anästhesie und Intensivtherapie, Klinikum
der Philipps-Universität, Marburg, Bundesrepublik Deutschland

Die respiratorische Insuffizienz umfaßt ein ausgedehntes Spektrum an Erkrankungen bei dem auf der einen Seite der normal ernährte fiebrige Patient mit einem ARDS und auf der anderen Seite der schlecht ernährte normotherme Patient mit einer chronisch obstruktiven Atemwegserkrankung (COPD) steht. Eine Standarderhährung, die alle pathophysiologisch-metabolischen Veränderungen innerhalb dieser doch recht inhomogenen Patientenpopulation berücksichtigt gibt es zwar nicht, doch kann die Frage nach der Notwendigkeit einer, auf die Bedürfnisse des respiratorisch insuffizienten Patienten abgestimmte Ernährung, die zudem den Erfordernissen der jeweiligen Krankheitsphase (kontrollierte Beatmung, asistierte Beatmung, Weaning, Spontanatmung) Rechnung trägt, grundsätzlich mit *JA* beantwortet werden. Diese Feststellung begründet sich wie folgt:

Ernährungsstatus und Funktion der respiratorischen Muskulatur

Die Häufigkeit eines Gewichtsverlustes bei Patienten mit einer beeinträchtigten Lungenfunktion – akut oder chronisch – wird in der Literatur mit 20–50 % angegeben. Besonders bei Patienten mit einer COPD stellt die allgemeine Auszehrung mit einer Reduktion des Körpergewichtes um mehr als 20 % des Sollwertes bis hin zu kachektischen Zuständen ein nicht ungewöhnliches Problem dar. Die Ursachen dafür finden sich in einer unzureichenden Energiezufuhr. Deshalb muß, unabhängig davon ob es sich um Patienten mit einer COPD oder um Patienten mit einer akuten respiratorischen Insuffizienz auf dem Boden von Sepsis, Trauma oder Verbrennung etc. handelt, die Energiezufuhr dem jeweiligen Bedarf angepaßt werden [7].

In diesem Zusammenhang finden sich unter ernährungsmedizinischen Gesichtspunkten grundsätzlich zwei Arten von Patienten in intensivmedizinischer Betreuung: 1. Patienten die wegen ihrer Grunderkrankung verbunden mit einer signifikanten Organstörung einen recht hohen Energieverbrauch aufweisen und bei denen deshalb ein hohes Risiko für eine Unterernährung besteht und 2. Patienten die bei der Aufnahme in die Intensivstation fehlernährt sind und die wegen ihres schlechten Ernährungsstatus für ernährungsbedingte Komplikationen, u. a. im Zusammenhang mit einer erneuten Exacerbation eines chronischen Infektes besonders anfällig sind. Patienten mit einer Fehlernährung und der Notwendigkeit zur maschinellen Ventilation hatten eine höhere Mortalität als beatmungspflichtige Patienten mit einem ausgeglichenen Ernährungsstatus [9].

Bei der Erfassung des Energieumsatzes ist die Gewichtskontrolle in der akuten Erkrankungsphase ungeeignet, da u. a. durch eine Katabolie Wasser freigesetzt und durch eine Überdruckbeatmung mit einem hohen intrathorakalen Druck eine Wasserretention begünstigt wird. Auch ist die Flüssigkeitsbilanz, unter Berücksichtigung der Tatsache, daß die Flüssigkeitsverluste oft nur unzureichend erfaßt werden können nur eingeschränkt beurteilbar. Zudem wird immer noch zu selten berücksichtigt, daß beispielsweise 1 l einer 25%igen Kohlenhydratlösung 845 ml Wasser enthält und 1 l einer 20%igen Fettlösung einen quantitativen Wassergehalt von 740 ml aufweist, was zusätzlich die Verwertbarkeit von Flüssigkeitsbilanzen einengt. Die Bestimmung des Energieumsatzes mit der Methode der indirekten Kalorimetrie ist zwar ein sehr gut geeignetes und mittlerweile auch durchführbares aber insgesamt immer noch aufwendiges Verfahren. Eine Beurteilung des Energieumsatzes durch Schätzwerte anhand standardisierter Algorithmen ist einfacher handhabbar, doch wird dabei der tatsächliche Energiebedarf des einzelnen Patienten leicht über- bzw. unterschätzt.

Eine Fehlernährung beeinträchtigt die thorakopulmonale Funktion auf 3 Ebenen:

Struktur und Funktion der respiratorischen Muskulatur

Im Hungerstoffwechsel dient als Energiequelle für den Organismus das Fettgewebe. Demgegenüber benutzt der kritisch Kranke hormonell bedingt, bes. dann wenn eine angemessene Energiezufuhr fehlt, Aminosäuren via Proteolyse und Glukoneogenese zur Energiegewinnung. Hält dieser Zustand an, so atrophieren, als Ausdruck eines gesteigerten Proteinkatabolismus die diaphragmalen, interkostalen und akzessorischen respiratorischen Muskeln, die aufgrund ihres hohen Proteingehaltes einen großen Anteil am Gesamteiweißbestand des Organismus darstellen [2]. Bei Patienten mit einem Lungenemphysem fanden sich insbesondere eine Atrophie der Zwerchfellmuskulatur, die stärker ausgeprägt war als bei untergewichtigen Patienten. Dementsprechend konnte bei Patienten mit einer COPD, die zudem einen Gewichtsverlust erlitten hatten, die Kraftentwicklung bei der Atemarbeit, darstellbar an verschiedenen dynamischen Lungenfunktionsparametern, als deutlich reduziert konstatiert werden. Eine signifikante positive Korrelation von „body cell mass" und maximaler inspiratorischer Kraft wurde nachgewiesen. Die herabgesetzte Zwerchfellfunktion bei Patienten mit einer akuten respiratorischen Insuffizienz wird durch eine gleichzeitig bestehende Hypophosphatämie perpetuiert. Eine Hypophosphatämie ist zudem immer ein Indikator für eine schlechte Ernährung und repräsentiert ein Mißverhältnis von Energiebedarf und Energiezufuhr [4].

Atemantrieb

Bei einer durch eine Fehlernährung bedingten Malnutrition mit konsekutiver Reduktion der Stoffwechselaktivität kommt es zu einer Verminderung des Atemantriebs. Besonders bei Patienten mit einer COPD kann dadurch ein respiratorisches Versagen begünstigt werden. Demgegenüber erhöht ein hohes Stickstoffangebot das AMV. Dabei sollte der Anteil der Aminosäure (AS) Tryptophan so gering wie möglich gehalten werden, da diese cerebral zu Serotonin, welches hemmend auf den Atemantrieb wirkt, umgebaut wird. Verzweigtkettige AS wiederum hemmen die Aufnahme von Trypotphan in das zentrale Nervensystem.

Immunsystem

Unter- und Fehlernährung führen zur Supression der Immunkompetenz und damit zu einer erhöhten Anfälligkeit für Infekte mit einer gesteigerten Morbidität und Mortalität. Dabei wurden vorwiegend Veränderungen in der zellulär-vermittelten Immunantwort nachgewiesen [8]. Auch wird von einer verminderten zellulären Resistenz der tracheobronchialen Mukosa gegenüber bakteriellen Infektionen bei unterernährten Patienten mit einem Tracheostoma berichtet. Zu den wesentlichsten Komplikationen bei einer akuten respiratorischen Insuffizienz gehören pulmonale Infektionen, speziell solche mit nosokomialer Genese die zu einem septischen Krankheitsbild führen können. Pneumonie und Spesis sind demzufolge auch die häufigsten Komplikationen bei fehlernährten kritisch kranken Patienten.

Wechselwirkungen der Nährsubstrate mit Stoffwechsel und Gasaustausch

Seit den Untersuchungen von Askanazi [3] ist der enge Zusammenhang von Stoffwechsel und pulmonaler Ventilation bekannt. Unter einer rein kohlenhydratorientierten Ernährung fand sich dabei ein erheblicher Anstieg der Kohlendioxidabgabe (VCO_2) mit der Notwendigkeit zu einer gesteigerten alveolären Ventilation. Bei der Durchführung einer totalen parenteralen Ernährung mit Glukose als alleinigem Energiedonator konnte bei Patienten mit einer Sepsis eine Erhöhung der VCO_2 um 57 % gegenüber einer zuvor stattgehabten hypokalorischen Ernährung mit einer 5%igen Glukoselösung beobachtet werden. Allerding stieg gleichzeitig auch die Sauerstoffaufnahme (VO_2)

um 30 % an, wodurch der respiratorische Quotient (RQ) niedriger als 1 bestimmt wurde [3]. Diese unter einer parenteralen Ernährung gewonnenen Erkenntnisse wurden durch Beobachtungen an enteral ernährten Patienten ergänzt [1]. Beim Vergleich von kohlenhydratreicher versus fettreicher Diät fanden sich dabei jedoch voneinander abweichende Ergebnisse. So konnte unter einer fettreichen Diät sowohl eine reduzierte als auch eine gleichbleibende VCO_2 abgebildet werden.

In einer eigenen Untersuchung an vollständig enteral ernährten gesunden Probanden die standardisiert sowohl kohlenhydratreich (50 % der Gesamtkalorien als Kohlenhydrate) als auch fettreich (50 % der Gesamtkalorien als Fett) ernährt wurden konnten wir eine signifikante Reduktion ($p < 0{,}001$) der VCO_2 unter der fettreichen Diät im Vergleich zur kohlenhydratreichen Diät beobachten. Hinsichtlich der VO_2 war zwischen den beiden Diäten zwar kein sicher signifikanter Unterschied darstellbar, doch fand sich unter der kohlenhydratreichen Diät ein deutlicher tendenzieller Anstieg der VO_2.

In einer kontrollierten Beobachtungsstudie an vollständig enteral ernährten Patienten mit einer ausgeprägten respiratorischen Insuffizienz und einem septischen Krankheitsbild, die entweder kohlenhydratreich (50 % der Gesamtkalorien) oder fettreich (50 % der Gesamtkalorien) ernährt wurden, untersuchten wir anhand der klinischen Parameter arterieller Kohlendioxidpartialdruck ($paCO_2$) und Atemminutenvolumen (AMV) den Einfluß der unterschiedlichen Substratzufuhr auf die Kohlendioxidbelastung dieser Patienten. Um den Schweregrad des jeweiligen Krankheitsbildes zu berücksichtigen erfolgte zudem eine Graduierung mit dem Sepsis-Score von Elebute und Stoner. Auch nachdem die Kontrollvariablen AMV und Score-Wert aus der abhängigen Variable $paCO_2$ mittels Kovarianzanalyse herauspartialisiert wurden zeigte sich, daß der unterschiedlich hohe Kohlenhydratanteil in der enteralen Ernährung keinen statistisch signifikanten Einfluß auf die Höhe des $paCO_2$ hatte (s. Abb. 1). Diese Ergebnisse stehen im Kontrast zu einer anderen Untersuchung [1] die eine Reduktion von $paCO_2$, AMV und Beatmungsdauer bei respiratorisch insuffizienten Patienten unter einer einen hohen Fettanteil aufweisenden enteralen Diät beschreibt.

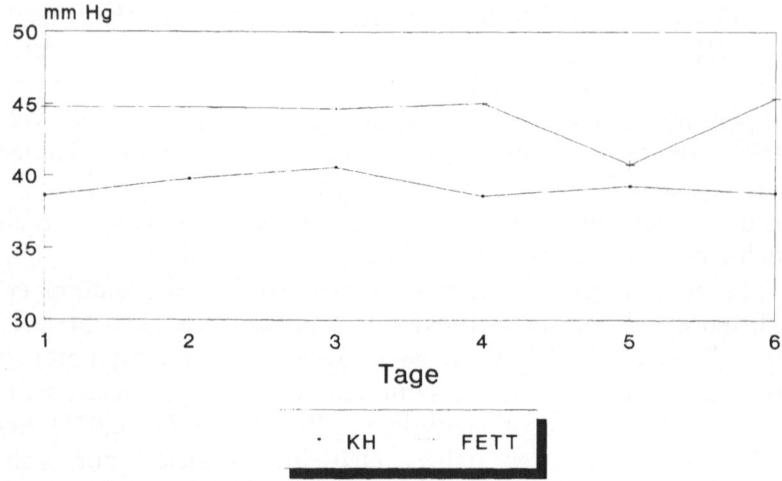

Abb. 1. Das Verhalten des Kohlendioxidpartialdrucks im arteriellen Blut (paCO$_2$) in Abhängigkeit von einer fettreichen (FETT) und einer kohlenhydratreichen (KH) Diät bei Patienten mit einer akuten respiratorischen Insuffizienz und septischem Krankheitsbild (s. Text)

In einer prospektiven Studie an 16 beatmungspflichtigen kritisch Kranken die bei vollständiger enteraler Nahrungszufuhr entweder eine kohlenhydratreiche (50 % der Gesamtkalorien; n = 8) oder eine fettreiche (50% der Gesamtkalorien; n = 8) Diät erhielten konnte der respiratorische Quotient (RQ) in der Gruppe der Patienten mit einer fettreichen Diät signifikant niedriger als in der Vergleichsgruppe bestimmt werden (Abb. 2). Dabei wurden die Patienten vor dem Beobachtungszeitraum schrittweise an die jeweilige Diät adaptiert, so daß zu Beginn der Untersuchung (Tag 1) bereits eine vollständige Umstellung auf die jeweilige Substratzusammensetzung erfolgt war. Dieses Ergebnis weist eindeutig auf eine geringere VCO$_2$ unter einer fettreichen Ernährung hin. Auch in dieser Studie fanden sich Hinweise auf eine Steigerung der VO$_2$ unter der kohlenhydratreichen Diät.

Auch wenn andere Arbeitsgruppen den Nutzen einer fettreichen Ernährung insbesondere bei akut respiratorisch insuffizienten Patienten relativieren und vielmehr darauf hinweisen, daß für diese Patienten die Sicherstellung einer be-

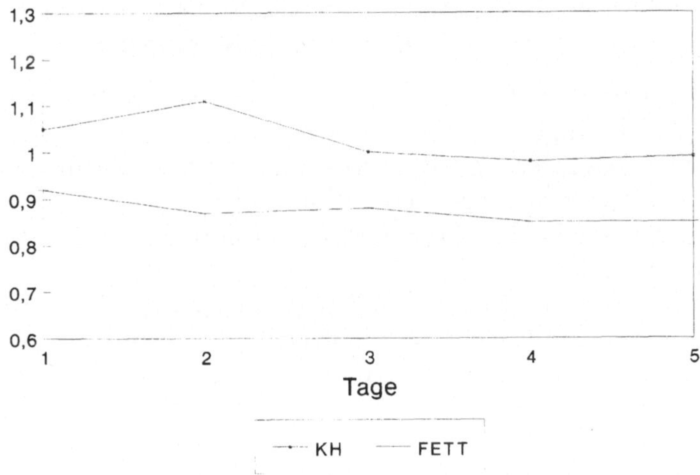

Abb. 2. Das Verhalten des respiratorischen Quotienten in Abhängigkeit von einer fettreichen (FETT) und einer kohlenhydratreichen (KH) Diät bei Patienten mit einer akuten respiratorischen Insuffizienz (s. Text)

darfsgerechten Zufuhr energieliefernder Substrate mit proteinsparender Wirkung eine sehr viel größere Relevanz hat, so muß doch zusammenfassend konstatiert werden, daß ein hohes Kohlenhydratangebot eine erhebliche Mehrproduktion von CO_2 bewirken kann und daß eine Reduktion des Kohlenhydratanteils zugunsten von Fett einen zumindest meßbaren Abfall der VCO_2 bewirkt.

Es ist jedoch unstrittig, daß Patienten mit einer COPD und einem reduzierten Ernährungszustand in ihrem Stoffwechselverhalten anders reagieren als kritisch Kranke mit einem konsekutiven Hypermetabolismus. So gibt es Hinweise darauf, daß bei den letztgenannten Patienten mit einem hohen Kohlenhydratangebot nicht nur die VCO_2 sondern auch die VO_2 ansteigt [3, s. o.]. Ein Abfall des RQ ist dann die logische Folge.

Bezüglich des bisher angenommenen größeren proteinsparenden Effekts der Kohlenhydrate [9] konnte durch die Analyse von Stickstoffbilanzen eine im Vergleich zu den Kohlenhydraten gleichwertige Wirkung der Fette auf den Proteinumsatz nachgewiesen werden [6].

Der Einfluß der Ernährung auf die Mediatoren und die Endothelzellen in der Lungenstrombahn

Die Kennzeichen des respiratorischen Versagens sind:

- Veränderungen im Gastaustausch von CO_2 und O_2 zwischen Alveolen und Blut, vor allem durch Störungen des Gleichgewichtes von Ventilation und Perfusion;
- Störungen in der Surfactantproduktion durch die Pneumocyten II;
- Alteration der Endothelzellen durch aus der Interaktion von Makrophagen und Neutrophilen Granulocyten mit den Endothelzellen freigesetzte Mediatoren und einer daraus resultierenden Änderung des Stoffwechsels dieser Zellen.

Die Endothelzellen in der Lungenstrombahn sind, insbesondere beim akuten Lungenversagen, metabolisch aktiv. So können sie einerseits Substanzen aufnehmen (z. B. Aufnahme von Serotonin und Propanolol) bzw. abbauen (z. B. Noradrenalin und Bradykinin) und andererseits, besonders auch durch den interzellulären Kontakt mit Neutrophilen Granulocyten und Makrophagen, Mediatoren (z. B. aktive Metabolite des Arachidonsäurestoffwechsels) freisetzen die zwar primär zu lokalen jedoch potentiell auch zu systemischen Effekten führen.

Neuere Studien geben Hinweise auf die Beeinflußbarkeit der pulmonalen Hämodynamik durch die intravenöse Zufuhr von Fettemulsionen. Durch Veränderungen im Ventilations/Perfusionsverhältnis kommt es zu einer Verschiebung im Verhalten des pulmonalen Gasaustausches. Dabei wird dieser Einfluß auf den pulmonalen Gefäßtonus allem Anschein nach durch Eicosanoide vermittelt, die aus den essentiellen Fettsäuren gebildet werden, und die sowohl Cyclooxygenaseprodukte als auch Lipoxygenaseprodukte der Arachidonsäure umfassen. Unklar ist jedoch nach welchen Regeln beispielsweise die agonistisch (z. B. PGE_2) und antagonistisch (z. B. PGF_{2alpha}) auf eine Vasodilatation in der Lungenstrombahn wirkenden Prostaglandine dabei gesteuert werden.

So konnten beispielsweise Suchner und Mitarbeiter [10] die Wirkung einer parenteralen Fettzufuhr auf die Lungenfunktion in Abhängigkeit von der Applikationsgeschwindigkeit und verschiedenen Grunderkrankungen (Sepsis versus ARDS) beobachten. Dabei fand sich unter einer schnellen Infusion (6 Stunden Applikationsdauer) bei einer Sepsis eine Reduktion des intrapulmonalen Shunts und eine Zunahme der Oxygenierung und beim ARDS eine erhöhte Shuntfraktion mit konsekutiver Abnahme des Quotienten paO_2/FIO_2, wohingegen die langsame Zufuhr über 24 Stunden insbesondere beim ARDS einen reduzierten intrapulmonalen Shunt mit einer günstigeren Sauerstoffaufnahme ermöglichte. Gasaustausch und Höhe der Shuntfraktion korrelierten dabei eng mit dem Quotienten $6\text{-Keto-PGF}_{1alpha}/TXB_2$.

Inwieweit eine Fettzufuhr die Bildung des Surfactant (Phosphatidylcholin, ein gesättigtes Lezithin, bildet eine Hauptkomponente pulmonaler Surfactant-Lipide) qualitativ bzw. quantitativ beeinflussen kann entzieht sich gegenwärtig noch einer abschließenden Beurteilung. Immerhin konnte bei traumatisierten Ratten durch eine intravenöse Fettzufuhr ein Anstieg der Lezitihin-Fraktion bewirkt werden der mit einer Verbesserung der Lungenfunktion dieser Tiere einherging [5].

Praktische Leitlinien für die Ernährung von Patienten mit einer respiratorischen Insuffizienz

Als Konsequenz aus den vorstehenden Erkenntnissen lassen sich gegenwärtig für den Patienten mit einer respiratorischen Insuffizienz nachfolgende „Eckpfeiler" für eine dem Krankheitsbild angepaßte Ernährung definieren:

- In der Akutphase einer respiratorischen Insuffizienz sollte eine restriktive Flüssigkeitszufuhr erfolgen (ca. 80–100 ml/h) und ggf. eine positive Flüssigkeitsbilanz durch die Gabe von Diuretika oder durch Hämofiltration abgebaut werden. In der Weaning-Phase kommt es zu einer Rückresorption von Flüssigkeit, so daß hier negative Bilanzen der Norm entsprechen.

- Die ausreichend hohe Dosierung von nichtprotein-Kalorien ist im Sinne einer bedarfsgerechten Energiezufuhr, insbesondere auch um einen Proteinkatabolismus zu verhindern unerläßlich.

– Durch die Bestimmung des Energieumsatzes (z. B. durch indirekte Kalorimetrie) und die tägliche Erstellung einer Stickstoffbilanz wird ein Ernährungsmonitoring zur Sicherstellung und Überwachung einer bedarfsgerechten Substratzufuhr herbeigeführt.

– Ein hohes Eiweißangebot, insbesondere in einer differenzierten Zusammensetzung, erhöht den Atemantrieb und reduziert die Aufnahme von Tryptophan in das zentrale Nervensystem. Dabei kann ein gesteigerter Atemantrieb therapeutisch sinnvoll jedoch auch schädlich sein. Ob die zu erwartende Wirkung einen unterstützenden Effekt hat hängt dabei vom individuellen Zustand des jeweiligen Patienten ab. Die empfohlene tägliche Dosierung wird dabei mit 1,5 g/kg KG angegeben und sollte in der Phase des Weaning ggf. reduziert werden.

– Bei der Kohlenhydratzufuhr ist eine Reduktion zugunsten von Fett besonders dann indiziert wenn eine Kohlendioxidbelastung vermieden werden soll, d. h. bei einer verminderten Ventilierbarkeit der Lunge, beim Weaning und in Fällen einer eingeschränkten pulmonalen Reserve sowie bei einer COPD. In diesen Fällen empfiehlt sich eine Anhebung des Fettanteils auf 50 % der Gesamtkalorien. Die Fettzufuhr sollte kontinuierlich über einen Zeitraum von 24 Stunden erfolgen und die Kontrolle der Triglyceridkonzentration im Serum unter laufender Zufuhr bedingen.

– Eine Hypophosphatämie ist zu vermeiden.

Literatur

1. Al-Saady MN, Blackmore CM, Benett ED (1989) High fat, low carbohydrate, enteral feeding lowers paCO$_2$ and reduces the period of ventilation in artifically ventilated patients. Intensive Care Med 15: 290

2. Amstrong JN (1986) Nutrition and the respiratory patient. Nutrition Supp Serv 6: 8

3. Askanazi JS, Rosenbaum J, Hyman AL, et al (1980) Respiratory changes induced by the large glucose loads of total parenteral nutrition. J Am Med Assoc 234: 1444

4. Aubier M, Murciano D, Lecogguic Y, et al (1985) Effects of hypophosphatemia on diaphragmatic contractility in patients with acute respiratory failure. N Engl J Med 313: 420

5. Bahrami S, Strohmaier W, Redl J, et al (1987) Mechanical properities of the lung of posttraumatic rats are improved by including fat in total parenteral nutrition. J Parenter Enteral Nutr 11: 560

6. Hayungs J, Michalzik V, Borchard F, et al (1987) Der Einfluß von Lipidemulsionen auf die Stickstoffbilanz im Rahmen eines peroperativen parenteralen Ernährungsregimes. Infusionstherapie 14: 23

7. Leong ET, Beno MC, Libby G (1983) Nutritional care of the ventilator-dependant patient: role of the dietitian. Nutrition Supp Serv 3: 7

8. McMurray D, Loomis S, Casazza L, et al (1981) Development of impaired ill-mediated immunity in mild and moderate malnutrition. Am J Clin Nutr 34: 68

9. Pingleton SK (1986) Nutrition in the acute respiratory failure. Lung 164: 127

10. Suchner U, Beck K, Katz DP, et al (1993) Einfluß parenteral verabreichter Fettemulsionen auf die Lungenfunktion. Akt Ernähr Med 18: 71

Korrespondenz: Dr. W. Höltermann, Abteilung für Anästhesie und Intensivtherapie, Klinikum der Philipps-Universität, Baldingerstraße, D-35043 Marburg, Bundesrepublik Deutschland

Spezielle Probleme bei der Entwöhnung vom Respirator

C. A. Zauner, A. Kranz, R. C. Apsner, L. Kramer, C. Madl,
K. Ratheiser, F. Stockenhuber, B. Schneeweiß und K. Lenz

Intensivstation, Klinik für Innere Medizin IV,
Universität Wien, Österreich

Viele kritisch Kranke bedürfen während ihres intensivstationären Aufenthaltes oder nach schwerwiegenden Operationen einer Atmungsunterstützung durch einen Respirator. Trotz Beherrschung der zugrundeliegenden Erkrankung, ausreichender Ernährung und einer allgemeinen klinischen Verbesserung wird ein signifikanter Anteil der Patienten für eine bestimmte Zeit respiratorabhängig. Die Inzidenz wird mit bis zu 20 % angegeben [1]. Das Unvermögen der Patienten eine ausreichende Spontanatmung aufrecht erhalten zu können, ist multifaktoriell. Die Ursachen eines respiratorischen Versagens sind entweder intrinsischer, wie zum Beispiel eine zugrundeliegende COPD, oder extrinsischer Natur, wie Deformitäten der Thoraxwand, ein verminderter zentralvenöser Atemantrieb oder eine Dysfunktion der Atemmuskulatur [2]. Sehr lange Respiratorunterstützung verursacht einen Schwund der Atemmuskulatur, Schwächung, rasche Ermüdbarkeit und sogar Atrophie.

Weaningkriterien

Die traditionell angewandten Weaningkriterien, wie Blutgasanalyse, Vitalkapazität, der mittlere inspiratorische Druck und Atemminutenvolumen wurden in letzter Zeit als zu ungenau erachtet, um ein erfolgreiches Entwöhnen vom Respirator voraussagen zu können [3, 5]. Einige dieser Patienten verfügen über eine so schlechte Atemmechanik, daß sie einen adäquaten Gasaustausch nicht aufrecht erhalten können. Andere wieder würden eine relativ gute Atemmechanik aufweisen; doch auch diese würden ohne Respirator keinen suffizienten Gasaustausch gewährleisten können [3]. Diese Patienten weisen möglicherweise einen verminderten zentralnervösen Atemantrieb auf, oder sie leisten eine so hohe Atemarbeit, die ihnen eine Spontanatmung über längere Zeit unmöglich macht.

Atemarbeit

Die Atemarbeit (WOB) kann als Sauerstoffverbrauch der Atemmuskulatur (Oxygen cost of breathing) definiert werden [4]. Dieser kann aus der Differenz des Gesamtsauerstoffverbrauches zwischen Spontanatmung und kontrollierter Beatmung (dVO_2) berechnet werden. Die Atemarbeit wird als Prozentzahl des dVO_2 während künstlicher Beatmung angegeben. Die Atemarbeit beatmungspflichtiger Patienten wurde als brauchbares Hilfsmittel beschrieben, ein erfolgreiches Weaning vorauszusagen [3–6].

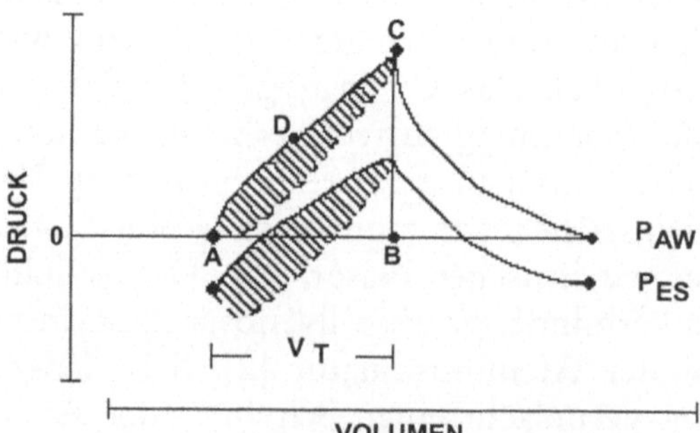

Abb. 1. (mod. nach Marini et al. [7]) Bestimmung der vom Patienten geleistete Atemarbeit (schematisch). Atemwegsdruck (P_{AW}) und Ösophagusdruck (P_{ES}) sind als Funktion der Lungenvolumsänderung unter kontrollierter (- - - - -) und assistierter (- - - -) Beatmung dargestellt. Die Fläche ABCDA stellt die vom Respirator geleistete Arbeit dar, wenn der Thorax passiv aufgeblasen wird. Die schraffierten Flächen zwischen den beiden Kurven ($P_{AW} \times V$ und $P_{ES} \times V$) repräsentieren die vom assistiert beatmeten Patienten geleistete Atemarbeit. Die beiden Kurven stellen zwei Möglichkeiten zur Bestimmung der Atemarbeit dar

Die gesamte mechanische Atemarbeit beatmeter Patienten setzt sich aus der physiologischen Atemarbeit plus der Atemarbeit zusammen, die durch das Beatmungsequipment und den Tubus (= breathing apparatus) verursacht wird. Die physiologische Atemarbeit muß zur Dehnung von Thoraxwand und Lungen durch ein bestimmtes Volumen geleistet werden.

Bestimmung der Atemarbeit

Die Bestimmung der mechanischen Atemarbeit kann anhand von Druck-Volumen-Kurven erfolgen. Die Atemarbeit entspricht der Fläche unter diesen Kurven (Abb. 1).

Unter kontrollierter Beatmung, wenn der relaxierte Thorax passiv von einem Respirator mit einem bestimmten Volumen aufgeblasen wird, kann jede dieser Komponenten berechnet werden.

$$W_{THX} = \int (P_{AW} - P_{ATM})\, Vdt = W_L + W_{CW}$$

$$W_L = \int (P_{AW} - P_{ES})Vdt$$

$$W_{CW} = \int (P_{ES} - P_{ATM})Vdt$$

(P_{AW} = Atemwegsdruck; P_{ATM} = Umgebungsdruck; P_{ES} = Ösophagusdruck; Vdt = Volumen pro Zeiteinheit)

W_{THX}, W_L, W_{CW} beschreibt die während der Inspirationsphase am Thorax, den Lungen und der Thoraxwand geleistete physiologische mechanische Arbeit.

Während assistierter Beatmung kann die W_L in ähnlicher Art und Weise berechnet werden. Doch weder die W_{CW} noch die W_{THX} kann anhand der oben dargestellten Gleichungen bestimmt werden.

$$W_L = \int P_{AW} - P_{ES})Vdt$$

$$W_{THX} = \qquad ?$$

$$W_{CW} = \qquad ?$$

Die vom Patienten geleistete mechanische Atemarbeit muß in indirekter Weise bestimmt werden. Dabei werden zwei Druck-Volumen-Kurven miteinander verglichen – einerseits unter voll kontrollierten Beatmungsbedingungen andererseits unter assistierten Bedingungen, wenn der Patient spontan triggert (Abb. 1).

Die Atemarbeit des breathing apparatus kann anhand folgender Gleichungen bestimmt werden:

$$W_{CIR} = \int PydV$$

= die Arbeit des Respirators, der Respiratorschläuche und der Verbindungsstücke. Dabei werden am Y-Stück der Respiratorschläuche die Druckänderungen und das Volumen gemessen.

Wenn diese beiden Größen am endotrachealen Tubusende gemessen werden (P_{ETT}), resultiert daraus die Atemarbeit des ganzen „breathing apparatus" (W_{APP}).

$$W_{APP} = \int P_{ETT}dV$$

Die vom Tubus verursachte Arbeit (W_{ETT}), errechnet sich aus der Differenz zwischen W_{APP} und W_{CIR}.

Sauerstoffverbrauch

Änderungen in der Arbeit, die vom Tubus alleine verursacht werden, ergeben sich aus der Interaktion von Innendurchmesser des Tubus und inspiratorischem Flow. Die Arbeit ist umgekehrt proportional zur Tubusgröße und direkt proportional zum Flow. Gemäß dem Gesetz nach Poiseuille ändern sich die Druckverhältnisse bei gleichbleibendem Flow mit der vierten Potenz des Tubusradius. Daraus ergibt sich ein steigender Atemwegswiderstand bei abnehmendem Tubusinnendurchmesser. Dies hat wiederum eine erhöhte Atemarbeit seitens der Patienten zur Folge. Diese vermehrte Atemarbeit verursacht ihrerseits einen erhöhten Sauerstoffverbrauch.

Der Sauerstoffverbrauch kann mittels zwei verschiedener Methoden bestimmt werden. Einerseits durch das Fick'sche Prinzip – dies allerdings setzt sehr invasive Interventionen mit ihren daraus erwachsenden Risiken voraus – andererseits durch die indirekte Kalorimetrie.

Bei kritisch Kranken kann der Sauerstoffverbrauch der Atemmuskulatur bis zu 50 % des Gesamtsauerstoffverbrauches einnehmen [5]. Unter diesen Voraussetzungen ist es natürlich nicht

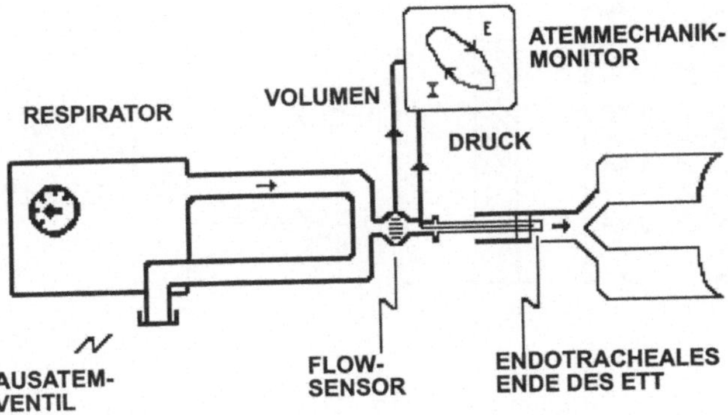

Abb. 2. Beatmungsequipment mit Beatmungsmonitoring (modifiziert nach Banner et al. [10])

möglich die Patienten erfolgreich vom Respirator zu entwöhnen. Für ein erfolgreiches Weaning finden sich in der Literatur verschiedene Angaben [3, 5, 8].

Kempter et al. [9] jedoch fanden keinen statistisch signifikaten Unterschied im Sauerstoffverbrauch zwischen erfolgreichen und erfolglosen Entwöhnungsversuchen. Nach Martin J. Tobin (1993) ist es unwahrscheinlich, daß die Messung der Atemarbeit als klinische Routinetechnik anerkannt wird, da relativ invasive und komplexe Messungen nötig sind.

Monitoring

Der in Abb. 2 dargestellte Bicore-Atemmechanikmonitor erlaubt eine Echtzeitanzeige der Druck-Volumen-Kurven und daraus die Berechnung der Arbeit, die vom breathing apparatus verursacht wird. Dabei wird die zusätzliche Arbeit als Integral aus Druck- und der Volumsänderung ausgedrückt. Der Druck wird hierbei am trachealen Ende des Tubus durch einen dünnen, luftgefüllten Katheter (1 mm Innendurchmesser) und die Volumsänderung durch einen kleinen Pneumotachographen (Flowsensor) bestimmt. Diese Methode erlaubt eine relativ rasche und unkomplizierte Messung der zusätzlichen Arbeit durch den breathing apparatus.

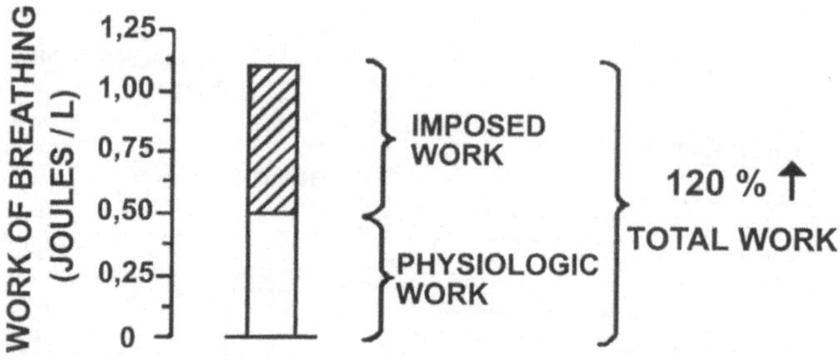

Abb. 3. (mod. nach Banner et al. [10]) Wenn man annimmt, daß die physiologische Atemarbeit 0,5 J/l (offener Anteil des Balkens), und die zusätzliche Atemarbeit weitere 0,6 J/l beträgt (schraffierter Anteil), resultiert daraus eine 120%ige Steigerung der gesamten Atemarbeit

Respiratorentwöhnung

Unter druckunterstützter Beatmung sollte die zusätzliche, durch das Beatmungsequipment verursachte Arbeit null sein, um die Nachlast der Atemmuskulatur soweit zu reduzieren, daß die gesamte Atemarbeit eher durch die Atemmechanik als durch die Widerstände und den breathing apparatus verursacht wird. Die Reduktion dieser zusätzlichen Arbeit auf null ist eine objektive, quantifizierbare und zielorientierte Richtlinie für die Anwendung der druckunterstützten Beatmung.

Die normale physiologische Atemarbeit für Erwachsene liegt etwa bei 0,5 J/l [11]. Banner et al. fanden eine zusätzliche Arbeit von 0,6 J/l mit einer Druckunterstützung von 0 mmHg. Das ergibt für einen Patienten in der Weaningendphase eine 120%ige Erhöhung der gesamten Atemarbeit (Abb. 3) [10].

Diese zusätzliche Atemarbeit erfordert eine Steigerung der Kontraktionskraft des Zwerchfells. Dies wiederum resultiert in einer erhöhten Atemarbeit, um die Spontanatmung aufrecht erhalten zu können. Patienten mit grenzwertiger Lungenfunktion und Muskelreserve, die sich von einem Lungenversagen erholen, können einer solchen Steigerung der Atemmuskelaktivität nicht standhalten. Diese Steigerungen der Atemarbeit führen zu einer Erhöhung des Sauerstoffverbrauches, zu einer raschen Ermüdung der Atemmuskulatur, Hyperkapnie und wiederum zu

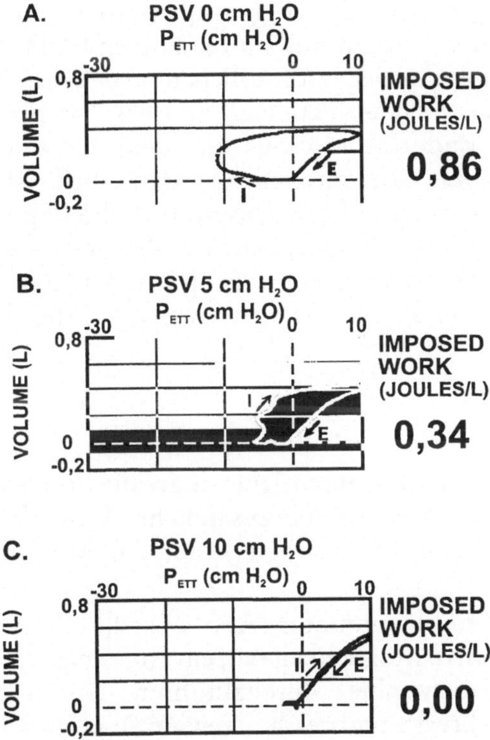

Abb. 4. (mod. nach Banner et al. [10]) Zusätzliche Atemarbeit bei **A** einem Druckniveau von 0 mmHg über PEEP, **B** einem Druckniveau von 5 mmHg über PEEP, **C** einem Druckniveau von 10 mmHg über PEEP. *PSV* pressure support ventilation; P_{ETT} Druck am endotrachealen Tubusende

einem neuerlichen respiratorischen Versagen. Das wiederum bedeutet eine Verlängerung der Intubationsdauer und predisponiert die Patienten wiederum für ein erhöhtes Risiko einer nosokomialen Infektion des Respirationstraktes.

Insuffiziente Druckniveaus schmälern die Effizienz der Atemmuskulatur und fördern die Muskelkraft auf Kosten der Muskelausdauer. Ein suffizientes Druckniveau ist nicht nur für die Patienten angenehmer, sondern fördert auch die Ausdauer der Atemmuskulatur. Es dürfte auch auf das Zwerchfell einen positiven Einfluß ausüben, das ein Paradebeispiel für einen primär auf Ausdauer ausgelegten Muskel darstellt.

Das Druckniveau, das ausgewählt werden sollte, um die zusätzliche Atemarbeit auf null zu reduzieren (Abb. 4), ergibt sich aus der Interaktion der erforderlichen inspiratorischen Flowrate eines spontanatmenden Patienten und des kombinierten Widerstandes von Endotrachealtubus und dem demand-flow System des Respirators. Die zusätzliche Atemarbeit ist direkt proportional dem erforderlichen inspiratorischen Spitzenfluß, dem Widerstand und der Ansprechzeit des demand-flow Systems des Respirators; es ist umgekehrt proportional zum Tubusinnendurchmesser und der Triggersensitivität des demand-flow Systems.

Schlußfolgerung

Es muß für jeden Patienten jenes individuelle Druckniveau gefunden werden, welches die zusätzliche Atemarbeit – und dadurch die gesamte Atemarbeit – auf ein Minimum reduziert (Abb. 4).

Der Atemmechanikmotor (Abb. 2) stellt eine relativ einfache und nichtinvasive Möglichkeit dar, ein Atemmechanikmonitoring direkt am Patientenbett durchzuführen. Durch die Echtzeitdarstellung – breath by breath – gewinnt man rasch einen Überblick über die zusätzliche Atemarbeit und andere atemmechanische Parameter beatmeter Patienten. Dadurch wird es möglich jederzeit das Druckniveau dem Patienten anzupassen, wenn die zusätzliche Atemarbeit ein tolerables Maß übersteigt.

Literatur

1. Tobin MJ, Perez W, Guenther SM, et al (1982) The pattern of breathing during successful and unsuccessful trials of weaning from mechanical ventilation. Am Rev Respir Dis 134: 1111
2. Roussos C, Macklem PT (1982) The respiratory muscles. N Engl J Med 307: 786
3. Fiastro LF, Habib MP, Shon BY, et al (1988) Comparison of standard weaning parameters and the mechanical work of breathing in mechanically ventilated patients. Chest 94: 232
4. Shikora SA, Bistrian BR, Borlase BC, et al (1990) Work of breathing: reliable predictor of weaning and extubation. Crit Care Med 18: 157

5. Lewis WD, Chwals W, Benotti PN, et al (1988) Bedside assessment of the work of breathing. Crit Care Med 16: 117
6. Marini JJ, Rodriquez RM, Lamb V (1986) Bedside estimation of the inspiratory work of breathing during mechanical ventilation. Chest 89: 56
7. Marini JM, Capps JS, Culver BH (1985) The inspiratory work of breathing during assisted mechanical ventilation. Chest 87: 612
8. Henning RJ, Shubin H, Weil MH, et al (1977) The measurement of the work of breathing for the clinical assessment of ventilator dependence. Crit Care Med 5: 264
9. Kemper M, Weissman C, Askanazi J, et al (1987) Metabolic and respiratory changes from mechanical ventilation. Chest 92: 979
10. Banner MJ, Kirby RR, Blanch PB, et al (1993) Decreasing imposed work of the breathing apparatus to zero using pressure-support ventilation. Crit Care Med 21: 1333
11. Otis AB (1964) The work of breathing. In: Fenn WO, Rahn H (eds) Handbook of physiology: a critical, comprehensive physiological knowledge and concepts. Section 3. Respiration. American Physiological Society, Washington DC, pp 463–476

Korrespondenz: Dr. Ch. A. Zauner, Intensivstation, Klinik für Innere Medizin IV, Universität Wien, Währinger Gürtel 18–20, A-1090 Wien, Österreich

Praktische Probleme der enteralen Ernährung

Vorgehen bei Reflux und bei Durchfall

J. M. Hackl

Klinik für Anästhesie und Allgemeine Intensivmedizin, Innsbruck, Österreich

Einleitung

Die enterale Ernährung hat in den letzten Jahren in der Behandlung von schwer kranken Menschen eine gewisse Bedeutung erlangt. Eine enterale Ernährung mit industriell gefertigten Diäten kann gerade beim Intensivpatienten zu Komplikationen führen und die enterale Ernährung ineffektiv machen. In der Literatur wird die Komplikationsrate bei dieser Form der Ernährung mit insgesamt bis zu 60% angesehen, sodaß die Sondenernährung dadurch vielfach in Mißkredit gerät.

Um die entsprechenden Komplikationen zu erkennen und entsprechend behandeln zu können, muß der Therapeut mit der Pathophysiologie der Ernährung beim schwer Kranken vertraut sein. Viele Voraussetzungen, die zur Veränderung der normalen Physiologie der Verdauung führen, wurden bereits in den Vorreferaten besprochen.

Folgende Komplikationen werden bei der Sondenernährung beschrieben (Abb. 1), hier sollen jedoch nur die für das Pflegepersonal bedeutendsten besprochen werden.

Reflux

Der postoperative Reflux wird zumeist als Ausdruck eines unvermeidlichen „postoperativen paralytischen Ileus" hin-

Art der Komplikation	Häufigk. [%]
Gastrointestinale Symptome	
– Reflux und „stille" Aspiration	20
– Diarrhöen	6-35
– Völlegefühl und Distensionen	10
– Obstipation	5
Metabolische Symptome	
– Hypertone Dehydration (Tube-feeding-Syndrom)	10
– Diabetische Stoffwechselstörungen	30
– Kardiale Dekomprensation	5
– Elektrolytveränderungen	25
– Mangel an essentiellen Fettsäuren u. Spurenelementen	?
– Transaminasenanstieg	20
Mechanische Komplikationen	
– Sondenverstopfung durch Diät	5
– Fehllage im Tracheobronchialsystem	<1
– Sonstige Sondendislokation	30
– Schleimhautläsionen (Pharynx, Ösophagus, Magen)	10
– Fremdkörpergefühl	
– Otitis media	
Infektionsprobleme	
– Aspirationspneumonie	2
– Bakterielle Kontamination	30

Abb. 1. Verschiedene Komplikationen der enteralen Sondenernährung

genommen und damit wird die nasogastrale Sonde prinzipiell indiziert. Untersuchungen über die Ursachen der gestörten Motilität in der postoperativen Phase sind zumeist schon älteren Datums und erst der zunehmende Einsatz der Sondenernährung hat dieses Problem wieder vordergründig werden lassen.

Interessant wurde der Reflux auch dadurch, daß man in den letzten Jahren in verschiedenen Studien nachweisen konnte, daß der Reflux von Mageninhalt nach Streß- ulcusprohylaxe mit H2-Antihistaminika gehäuft zu schweren Pneumonien führt.

Ein Reflux tritt bei der enteralen Ernährung von Intensivpatienten relativ häufig auf und ist nicht immer die Folge der Sondenernährung. In der Literatur wird die Häufigkeit eines Refluxes bei Sondennahrung mit Werten zwischen 10% und 50% angegeben. Um diese Zahlen besser interpretieren zu können, sollen die Ergebnisse einer an unserer Klinik durchgeführten Studie herangezogen werden.

Bei 104 Patienten der eigenen Intensivstation wurde das Reflux- und Stuhlverhalten unter enteraler Ernährung untersucht. Die Patienten wurden aufgrund ihrer Primärerkrankung in drei Gruppen unterteilt. Gruppe I beinhaltete polytraumatisierte Patienten mit Rippenserienfrakturen, Lungenkontusionen, Becken- und Extremitätenfrakturen, jedoch ohne Mitbeteiligung des Abdomens und Schädels. In der Gruppe II befanden sich Patienten mit einem Schädel-Hirn-Trauma und in der Gruppe III Patienten mit einem Polytrauma, bei denen es zusätzlich zu abdominellen Verletzungen gekommen war und die laparomiert werden mußten. Bei allen Patienten wurde unmittelbar nach der Aufnahme an der Intensivstation eine weitlumige Magensonde gelegt, die primär zur Drainage des Mageninhaltes diente, sekundär aber für die enterale Ernährung herangezogen wurde. Der Ernährungsaufbau erfolgte bei allen Patienten primär parenteral, anschließend wurde langsam auf eine niedermolekulare Diät umgestellt, wobei in der Gruppe III die parenterale Ernährung in einem höheren Ausmaß und bis zu einem längeren Zeitpunkt fortgeführt werden mußte. Die Osmolalität der niedermolekularen Diät betrug anfänglich durch entsprechende Verdünnung ca. 450 mosmol/l und wurde dann auf ca. 600 mosm/l gesteigert. Die Umstellung auf eine hochmolekulare nährstoffdefinierte Diät war in der Gruppe I und II vergleichbar, während eine Umstellung in der Gruppe III nur langsam durchgeführt werden konnte und in Einzelfällen wurde die Sondenernährung bis zum Abschluß des Untersuchungszeitraumes mit einer CDD durchgeführt.

Das Auftreten eines Refluxes und die Refluxmengen in den einzelnen Gruppen unterschieden sich in den ersten Tagen, d. h. vor Einsetzen der enteralen Nahrungszufuhr nicht voneinander, d. h. im Mittel kam es bei ca. 45% der Patienten

J. M. Hackl

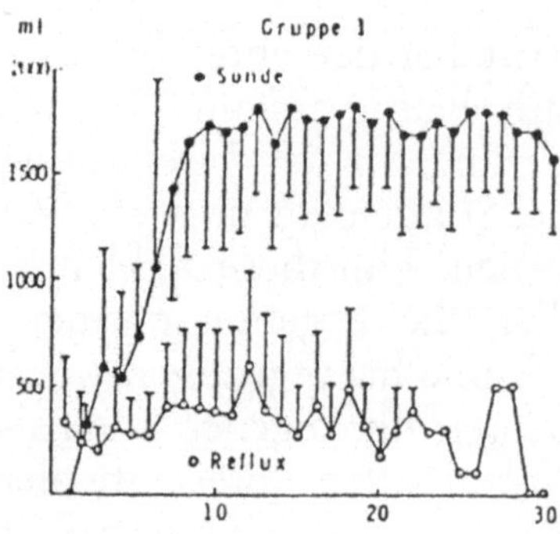

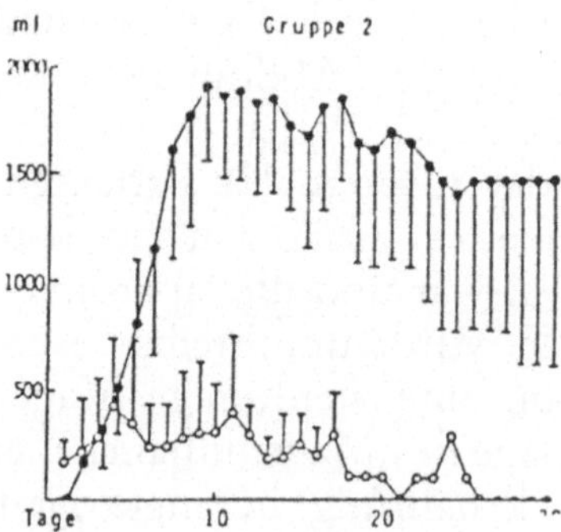

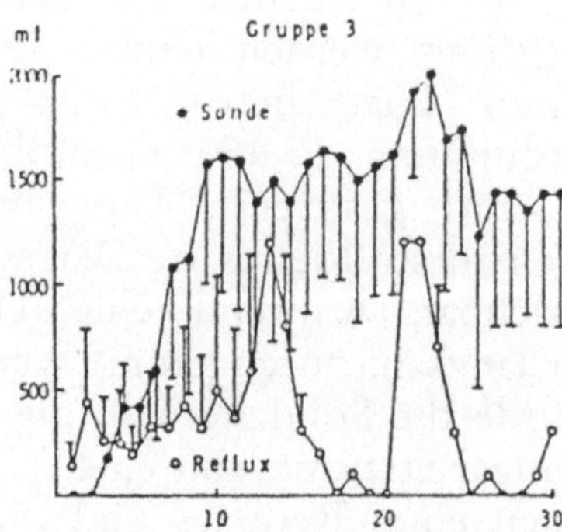

Abb. 2. Refluxverhalten bei den einzelnen Patienten und Ausmaß des Refluxes in den drei Untersuchungsgruppen

zu einem Reflux (Abb. 2). In den folgenden Untersuchungsperioden kam es zu einem steten Rückgang der Patienten mit Reflux, in der Gruppe III, bei den Patienten mit Abdominalverletzungen zeigte sich jedoch häufiger ein Reflux, obwohl die Sondenzufuhr langsamer und weniger bedarfsdeckend erfolgte. Die Menge des Refluxes nahm bei den Patienten der Gruppe I und II, die einen Reflux aufwiesen, zuerst noch zu, fiel dann aber stetig ab, die Patienten der Gruppe III zeigten im gesamten weiteren Verlauf relativ hohe Refluxmengen. Die Häufigkeit und die Höhe des Refluxes in der ersten Behandlungszeit mag darauf hinweisen, daß der Reflux nicht allein von der Sondennahrung abhängt und daß zu Beginn der Behandlung fast alle Patienten einen Reflux aufweisen.

Die Ursachen für den erhöhten Reflux sind vielfältig (Abb. 3). Hauptsächlich dafür verantwortlich ist die verzögerte Entleerung, die durch die neuromuskuläre Umstellung bei diesen Patienten bedingt ist, aber auch die Sonde selbst begünstigt das Auftreten eines Refluxes. Der Magenfundus hat die Fähigkeit, sich unterschiedlichen Füllungsvolumina so anzupassen, sodaß sich der Mageninnendruck nur wenig ändert. Diese rezeptive bzw. adaptative Relaxation wird durch inhibitorische Vagusfasern vermittelt und bewirkt, daß sich

---

Motilitätsstörungen („postoperativer Ileus")
- gestörte MMC
- medikamentös (Dopamin)

technische Probleme
- zu tiefe Sondenlage
- inadäquater Beginn
- inadäquate Sondenmenge
- inadäquate Zufuhrrate
- inadäquate Temperatur
- Patient liegt zu flach

Abb. 3. Ursachen des sondenbedingten Refluxes

der intragastrale Druck bei unterschiedlichen Füllungsvolumina nicht wesentlich ändert und es nicht zum Regurgi-
tieren kommt. Durch ein Trauma, durch Eingriffe in den Ga-
strointestinaltrakt, retroperitoneale Hämatome kommt es zu
einer direkten Störung der Motilität oder zu einem Überwiegen des Sympathikus und damit zur Aufhebung der Kon-
stanz des Mageninnendruckes, der Mageninhalt wird vermehrt regurgitiert. Dies zeigt sich besonders in der Gruppe III
der untersuchten Patienten. Zusätzlich haben Anästhetika
und Sedativa (z. B. Thiobarbiturate) dosisabhängig einen
direkten Einfluß auf den Tonus und die Motilität des Magens.
Aus der lokalen Störung, dem Überwiegen des Sym-
pathikotonus und der Wirkung verschiedener Pharmaka resultiert das Bild der „postoperativen Darmatonie". Der Py-
lorus zeigt zudem vielfach einen erhöhten Tonus, wobei auch
vielfach ein duodeno-gastraler Reflux zu beobachten ist.
Durch die Erhöhung des Druckgradienten kommt es zu
einem Rücklauf der Nahrung und damit zum Reflux.

Die Entleerung von Nahrung verschiedener Konsistenz ist
primär eine Funktion des Druckgradienten. Bei Intensivpatienten zeigt sich, daß bei der Bolusapplikation die Refluxmengen zumeist größer sind, eine eindeutige Abhängigkeit
konnte bei unseren Patienten nicht festgestellt werden.

Zahlreiche weitere Faktoren, die durch die Nahrung bedingt sind, bestimmen die Entleerungsgeschwindigkeit
(Abb. 4). Hierzu zählen Volumen und Beschaffenheit des Mageninhaltes wie Azidität, Osmolarität, Energiekonzentration
sowie Gehalt an langkettigen Fettsäuren und Tryptophan,
wobei Rezeptoren im Duodenum und Jejunum dafür verantwortlich sind: ein hyperkalorischer Mageninhalt hemmt
z. B. die Magenentleerung. Auch die Osmolarität beeinflußt
die Entleerung des Magens ebenfalls durch spezifische Rezeptoren im Duodenum und Jejunum.

Daneben beeinflussen zahlreiche Erkrankungen die Magenentleerung; im allgemeinen wird sie verzögert. Als Beispiele
seien angeführt: die diabetische Gastroparese, die Vagotomie
und die Dysrhythmie des Magens.

Ein Reflux ist bei intubierten, tracheotomierten und kontrollierten Patienten von besonderer Bedeutung, da es bei

Rezeptoren	Duodenum		Jeunum
	oral	aboral	
Dehnungsreiz	+	?	+
Osmorezeptoren	–	–	+
Säuren	+	–	+
Fette (C_{10}–C_{14})	–	–	+
Tryptophan	+	+	+

Abb. 4. Faktoren der Nahrungszusammensetzung, die die Magenentleerung beeinflussen

diesen gehäuft zu Aspirationen kommen kann. Die Aspirationen können wiederum zu schweren Pneumonien und zur Sepsis führen, da die Sondennahrung vielfach kontaminiert ist. Die Sondennahrung führt auf Grund ihrer Zusammensetzung zudem zu einem guten Keimwachstum, daneben ist der pH-Wert der Sondennahrung zu beachten. Eine Aspiration kann auch bei abgeblockten Tubus erfolgen und wird vielfach übersehen, die Komplikationen sind umso schlimmer. Die Aspiration ist das Hauptproblem des Refluxes bei der Sondenernährung.

Um eine Aspiration zu verhindern ist die Beachtung und Behandlung des Refluxes von besonderer Bedeutung. Da es an den ersten Behandlungstagen prinzipiell zu einer erhöhten Refluxmenge kommt, sollte mit der Sondenernährung erst dann kommen, wenn die Refluxmenge unter 500 ml/Tag beträgt. Bleibt diese weiterhin erhöht und können Faktoren, die durch die Nahrungszusammensetzung oder durch die Verhältnisse des Magen-Darm-Traktes bedingt sind, ausgeschlossen werden, so ist die Gabe eines Metoclopramid- oder Cisaprid-Derivates (Dopaminantagonisten) indiziert, dadurch können neuro-vegetative Einflüsse ausgeschalten werden. Die Sondenernährung selbst hat vielfach einen stimulierenden Effekt auf die Darmmotilität. Bessert sich der Reflux unter dieser Therapie nicht, so ist eine Nahrungskarenz einzuführen. Eine solche ist jedoch umstritten, da dadurch der

propulve Effekt der Nahrung verloren geht. Meist sind aber
Ursachen, die in der Applikation liegen, für den Reflux verantwortlich. Dies sind, daß die Sonde nicht richtig liegt (im
Ösophagus oder duodenal), die zugeführte Nahrungsmenge
zu kalt oder nicht richtig konzentriert ist und die Sondenmenge für den jeweiligen Zustand nicht entsprechend dosiert
ist. Diese Ursachen sollten in jedem Fall ausgeschalten werden.

Diarrhoen

Diarrhoen werden im Rahmen der enteralen Ernährung
häufig beschrieben und sind deshalb von besonderem Interesse, weil sie die Durchführung der Ernährung vielfach er-
schweren. Die Definition ist vielfach uneinheitlich, ob das
hier vorgestellte Score-System eine Verbesserung bringt, wird
sich zeigen (Abb. 5).

Um die Problematik der Diarrhoen zu verdeutlichen, soll
unsere vorher erwähnte Studie nochmals werden. Die erste
Defläkation trat zwischen dem 2. und 4. Behandlungstag auf.
Die Stuhlfrequenz nahm in allen Gruppen mit der Behand-
lungsdauer zu. Durchfälle traten an insgesamt 9 Tagen bei
7 Patienten im Verlauf von 1764 Behandlungstagen auf, dies
ist bei 6,7% der Patienten. In der Literatur werden vielfach
höhere Werte angegeben.

Die pathophysiologischen Mechanismen der Diarrhoen
liegen in folgenden Ursachen (Abb. 6):
– Die osmotische Ursache wird z. T. überbewertet. Bei zwei
  eigenen Untersuchungen mit Sondennahrungen unter-

Konsistenz	Geschätztes Volumen		
	< 200	200–250	> 250
Geformt	1	2	3
Breiig	3	6	9
Flüssig	5	10	15

Abb. 5. Diarrhoe-Score (nach Hart 1988)
„Diarrhoe" = Score × Stuhlfrequenz > 12/Tag

schiedlicher Osmolarität (500 mosmol gegenüber 310 mosmol) konnte kein signifikanter Unterschied im Auftreten von Diarrhoen vorgefunden werden. Zu Störungen durch die Osmolarität dürfte es hauptsächlich dann kommen, wenn die Nahrungsbestandteile nicht entsprechend resorbiert werden können. Dies zeigt sich besonders bei hohem Fettanteil, wo es durch die Fettmaldigestion zur osmotischen Diarrhoe kommt. Ein ähnlicher Effekt ist bei der Zufuhr von Laktose zu beobachten, jedoch wird Laktose bei den heutigen Nährstoffsubstraten kaum mehr verwendet.

– Inwieweit der Mangel an Natrium in der Sondennahrung bei der Diarrhoe mitspielt, ist noch ungeklärt, jedoch sprechen einzelne Untersuchungen dafür. Der Natriumgehalt der verschiedenen Substrate liegt z. T. unter 50 mmol/

Ursachen der sondenbedingten Diarrhoen:

osmotische Ursache
- niedermolekulare Nährsubstrate
- Elektrolyte (Natriumgehalt)
- Laktose

sekretorische Ursache
- Enterotoxine und bakterielles Overgrowthing
- gastrointestinale Hormone, Prostaglandine
- Laxantien

direkte Schleimhautschädigung
- hypoxische Schädigung und Reperfusion
- Freie Radikale

Motilitätsstörungen
- Störungen der MMC

medikamentöse Begleittherapie
- Antibiotika

Fehlen der Ballaststoffe

Abb. 6. Pathophysiologische Mechanismen der Diarrhoen

1000 kcal und hier vor allem leicht aufschließbaren Kohlenhydraten und kann zu Resorptionsstörungen von Kohlenhydraten führen, sodaß es wiederum zur osmotischen Diarrhoe kommt. Ein Auflösen von pulverförmiger Sondennahrung in physiologischer Kochsalzlösung kann die Diarrhoerate vermindern.

– Das Auftreten einer sekretorischen Diarrhoe wird durch Enterotoxine, durch gastrointestinale Hormone, durch Laxantien und andere Faktoren propagiert. Durch die gestörte Darmmotilität kommt es zu einer Überwucherung der Dünndarmflora mit lokalisationsfremden Keimen und in deren Folge durch die Endotoxine vermittelt zur sekretorischen Diarrhoe. Aber auch verschiedene gastrointestinale Hormone, die inadäquat ausgeschüttet werden, verursachen eine Hypersekretion in das Darmlumen. Inwieweit hier die Prostaglandine mitspielen, ist noch ungeklärt.

– Die Schleimhautschädigung ist ein gewichtiger Faktor bei der postoperativen bzw. posttraumatischen Ernährung. Die Darmschleimhaut ist gegenüber exogenen Noxen außerordentlich sensibel und der Darm gehört auf Grund seiner labilen Blutversorgung zu den sogenannten Schockorganen. In der Phase der Minderperfusion kommt es auch zur Schädigung des Epithels und Peroxide führen zu einem weiteren Untergang der Epithelzellen. Die Untersuchungen am Schockorgan „Darm" befinden sich noch im Anfangsstadium, weitere Untersuchungen werden hier Klarheit schaffen.

– Die Motilitätsstörungen wurden bereits beim Reflux angesprochen. Die Störung der MMC durch das Trauma im Sinne der „postoperativen Darmatonie", die Veränderungen der „Slow waves" und die gestörte Colonmotorik aggravieren diese Veränderungen. Einen zusätzlichen Einfluß ergeben die iatrogenen Maßnahmen wie Dopamingabe, Sedativa und Analgetika, Diuretika und Calciumantagonisten. Die Motilitätsfaktoren werden auch durch den Applikationsmodus beeinflußt. Eine zu rasche Verabfolgung der Sondennahrung, d. h. im Bolus, und zu große Mengen besonders bei Duodenal- und Jejunalsonden führen häufig zu Diarrhoen. Hier muß immer darauf geachtet werden, wo die Sondenspitze liegt. Gastrale bzw. duodenale Sondenapplikationen bedingen einen unterschiedlichen Applikationsmodus. Duodenal und jejunal soll nur eine kontinuierliche Zufuhr erfolgen, während bei gastraler Zufuhr die Bolusernährung gewisse Vorteile besitzt. Nachahmung des natürlichen Ernährungsverhaltens, bessere hormonelle Adaptation, geringeres thermodynamisches Äquivalent. Auch zu kalte Nahrung kann zu Veränderung der Darmmotilität und damit zu Diarrhoen führen.

– Eine medikamentöse Begleittherapie ist vielfach die Ursache von Diarrhoen, wobei hier besonders die Verabreichung von Antibiotika zu erwähnen ist.

– Der Einfluß von Ballaststoffen in der Ernährung kritisch Kranker wird kontroversiell behandelt. In der Primärphase bei Bestehen neurovegetativer Motilitässtörungen können Ballaststoffe vermehrt zu Diarrhoen führen, während diese bei der Langzeittherapie einen sehr positiven Effekt ausüben können.

Um Diarrhoen effizient verhindern zu können und deren Auftreten primär hintanzuhalten, ist es notwendig, die Ursachen dafür zu kennen und zu erkennen. Es muß bei jedem Auftreten von Diarrhoen nach dem auslösenden Faktor gesucht werden. Prinzipiell sollte bei Auftreten von Diarrhoen, soferne sie nicht durch die Applikation von Diarrhoika bedingt sind, die Sondennahrung für ca. 12 bis 24 Stunden abgesetzt werden, in der Zwischenzeit kann Tee angeboten werden. Nach Ausschalten der Ursache kann der Sondenaufbau wieder begonnen werden. Vielfach muß wiederum auf eine niedermolekulare Sondendiät umgestellt werden, um die Resorptionskapazitäten besser auszuschöpfen, und der Nahrungsaufbau muß wieder langsam gesteigert werden. In manchen Fällen wirkt sich die Zugabe von Pektin positiv aus. Der Patient muß in dieser Phase besonders genau monitiert werden und eventuelle Flüssigkeits- oder Energiedefizite müssen parenteral ausgeglichen werden.

Auf die anderen Komplikationsmöglichkeiten wie Fehllage der Sonde, Sondenverstopfung, Otitis media, Druckulcera und metabolische Störungen mit Hyperglykämie und Tube feeding Syndrom möchte ich hier nicht eingehen, sie sollen jedoch immer wieder in Erinnerung gerufen werden.

Die enterale Nahrungszufuhr besitzt aber andererseits einen schleimhautprotektiven Effekt, der die Barriere zwischen Darminnerem und dem endogenen Abwehrsystem aufrechterhält. Bei ausschließlicher parenteraler Ernährung kommt es schon nach wenigen Tagen zu einem Zusammenbrechen der Bakterienschranke der Darmmukosa und Keime der Darmflora können so in die Blutbahn gelangen. Dieser Weg der endogenen Infektion wird heute vielfach als Hauptursache der Sepsis bei Intensivpatienten angesehen. Untersuchungen der letzten Zeit haben auch gezeigt, daß eine adäquate Ernährung der Reifung der Lymphozyten beschleunigt.

Zusammenfassung

Der Einfluß von Operations- bzw. Traumastreß und der Medikation mit verschiedenen zentral und peripher wirksamen Substanzen führt zu einer bedeutsamen Dysbalance der Magenmotilität und damit zum verstärkten Reflux und zu Diarrhoen bes. in den ersten Tagen nach dem akuten Ereignis. Daneben haben die Nahrungszusammensetzung und verschiedene andere lokale und systemische Faktoren einen Einfluß auf die Verdauung. Eine Beeinflußung kann hier hauptsächlich durch Normalisierung der nervalen Störung (medikamentös, Periduralanästhesie usw.) erzielt werden. Der Einfluß der Nahrungszusammensetzung ist ebenfalls von großer Bedeutung (Applikationsart, Energiedichte, Osmolarität, pH-Wert, Natriumgehalt, Proteinzusammensetzung) und es ist darauf zu achten, daß bei der angebotenen Nahrung die oben beschriebenen Triggerfunktionen nach Möglichkeit ausgeschalten werden.

(Literatur beim Verfasser)

Korrespondenz: Prof. Dr. J. M. Hackl, Intensivstation, Klinik für Anästhesiologie und Allgemeine Intensivmedizin, Anichstraße 35, A-6020 Innsbruck, Österreich

Autorenverzeichnis

K. Lenz, P. G. H. Metnitz (eds.)

Patient Data Management in Intensive Care

1993. 24 figures. VII, 150 pages.
Soft cover DM 49,–, öS 350,–
ISBN 3-211-82513-4

(Intensivmedizinisches Seminar, Band 6)

Recent technological innovations - influenced primarily by the development of more sophisticated, faster and cheaper computer systems - permitted also the evolution of more affordable systems for Patient Data Management, so called PDM-Systems. The experience of the authors, on one of the first PDMS installation sites in Europe, shows that the purchase of such a system is not an easy task, since accurate data are not available in a comparable format. Therefore the first part of the book is devoted to a comparison of already installed, commercially distributed bedside based PDMS with regard to their specifications, functions and performance. The methods included a questionnaire with detailed questions for the vendors to answer and a "table of functions" comparing the most important functions which should be included in a PDMS. With that list the different systems (which were all in clinical use) were checked for the availability and the way of use of these functions. To evaluate variations in the systems performance an "information retrieval test" was designed and executed. In the second part the different vendors, whose systems were included in the study, were to describe the systems from their viewpoints. The third part contains papers describing the users' experiences. The fourth and last part shows how to use PDMS-data for scientific and therapeutic purposes including two papers on clinical expert systems. Thus, this book provides valuable information for clinicians and hospital managers who have to decide on the purchase of a Patient Data Management System.

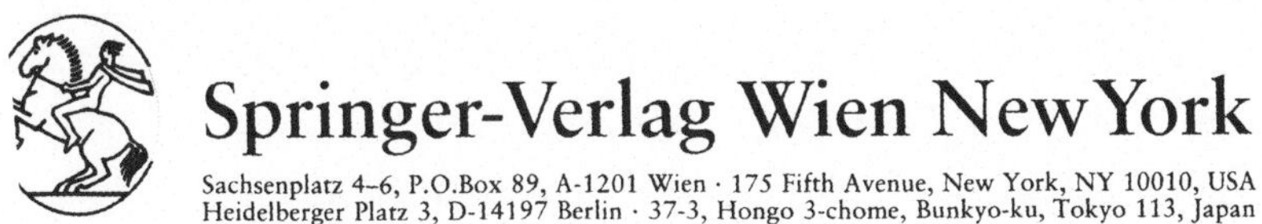

Springer-Verlag Wien New York

Sachsenplatz 4–6, P.O.Box 89, A-1201 Wien · 175 Fifth Avenue, New York, NY 10010, USA
Heidelberger Platz 3, D-14197 Berlin · 37-3, Hongo 3-chome, Bunkyo-ku, Tokyo 113, Japan